Documentation
in a SNAP

For Activity Programs

(Third Edition)

By
Ann G Uniack, RHIA

S N A P, Inc

(Skilled Nursing Assessment Programs)
P.O. Box 574
San Anselmo, CA 94979

Third Edition

First Printing May 2005
Second Printing July 2007

Printed in the United States of America

Published by: S. N. A. P., Inc. (Skilled Nursing Assessment Programs), P. O. Box 574, San Anselmo, CA 94979. Additional copies of this book may be ordered from the publisher. Prepaid orders only. Checks may be made payable to S N A P in the amount of $38.95 for each book, plus $4.00 shipping and handling. In California, please add sales tax of 7.75% ($3.02) per book.

ISBN: 978-1-881671-26-8

S N A P is the trademark of S.N.A.P., Inc.
Documentation in a SNAP is the trademark of a series of publications written by
Ann G Uniack

ABOUT THE AUTHOR

Ann G Uniack is a registered health information administrator. She has specialized in clinical record systems for skilled nursing facilities for more than twenty-five years. She is the principal consultant in a health information management firm providing services to nursing facilities in the San Francisco Bay Areas. Originally from Portland, Oregon, she received her Bachelor of Science in Medical Records Science from Seattle University.

Her professional activities have included election to Director of the California Health Information Association and President of the San Francisco Health Information Association. She has also served as committee chairman and member of various local, state and national professional association committees. She has been honored by the California Health Information Association as their Distinguished Member of the year.

Articles written by Ann G Uniack have been regularly published in the <u>CHIA Journal</u>. She is often a speaker at seminars on subjects such as documentation in the clinical record and ICD-9-CM coding.

Write it concise

Never write it twice

Table of Contents

Introduction

Charting is never a SNAP! And it is often a low priority. An activity professional's first interest is working with people. And rightly so.

Energy is directed toward improving the quality of life for residents in the nursing facility. Each resident has special needs. Success is measured by positive outcomes of care. To achieve positive outcomes, the interdisciplinary team must coordinate a plan of care that is right for each resident.

The purpose of this book is to create a system of documentation that supports the delivery of resident care. The clinical record provides the activity professional with information to:

- assess each resident's needs,

- develop a plan of care,

- establish goals to be achieved and outcomes expected,

- document interventions and

- evaluate the success or need for revision of the care plan.

Throughout this book there are references specific to the activity program in a nursing facility. Included within the chapters are sections from federal regulations with interpretive guidelines and the <u>Long Term Care Resident Assessment Instrument User's Manual</u> that apply to activity programs. *One can't play the game without knowing the rules.*

Information is the key to meeting residents' needs. Health professionals turn to the clinical record for that information. For the record to be useful, accurate and easy to find documentation must be available for staff to make decisions for resident care.

In other words, DOCUMENTATION must be a SNAP !

Clinical Record Guidelines

```
KEY POINTS AND SUMMARY OF CHAPTER

The clinical record is a legal document that is evidence of resident care.

Documentation in the clinical record must follow the rules for recording
in a legal document.

All resident information is organized and maintained in the clinical
record to allow easy access for all health care providers.

Resident health information is protected from loss, tampering or unau-
thorized access.
```

A. Legal Document

The clinical record is a business record. Records made in the regular course of business and at the time an event occurred are legal documents. Documentation in the clinical record is completed by members of the interdisciplinary team who have knowledge of the acts, events, conditions, opinions, or diagnoses concerning the resident. The clinical record is the evidence of the care that was given.

There are four requirements that must be met for the clinical record to be considered as evidence by of Court of Law.

- The record was documented in the normal course of business.

- The record was written at or near the time care was given.

- A person with knowledge of the resident's care wrote the documentation in the record.

- The record was stored in a safe and secure manner to prevent loss, tampering or unauthorized use.

When a health care professional completes clinical record documentation in a timely manner, that information is presumed to be true. A Court of Law considers the clinical record as the proof of work performed. It is often said, *If it was not documented, it was not done.*

A health care professional may sign a time sheet or punch a time clock to prove that he or she was present at work. But what is the proof that the person provided care to any residents?

The proof is the documentation in the clinical record, such as assessments, progress notes, attendance records and flow sheets of one-to-one visits. If documentation is not complete, there is no proof that a person has done his or her job. When records are not completed on time, the information can become suspect. An accurate clinical record is the best proof of care.

B. Rules for Recording

Because the clinical record is a legal document that is evidence of care, it is maintained according to approved facility procedures and state and federal regulations. There are rules for recording in legal documents that must be followed. If the rules for recording are not followed, the clinical record will not be considered accurate or true.

For example, consider documents that are handled in one's daily life. Credit card receipts and personal checks are legal documents. The person in possession of those documents can expect to be paid or to be obligated to pay the amount that is stated on the paper. These documents are business records completed in the regular course of business according to rules for recording on legal documents.

Now think about the clinical record. The clinical record is a legal document. It is proof that care was provided to the resident. It is evidence of the kind and quality of care given to a resident. The same principles that are used to write a check or complete a credit card transaction apply to the clinical record. Carefully follow the rules for recording to make sure that your documentation is legal.

1. Legible

The entries in the clinical record must be clearly written so other health care professionals can understand the entry. Often handwritten notes are made hastily and errors occur, which then are not corrected in a legible manner. Or staff may use abbreviations as a shorthand. Allow enough time to make thoughtful and clear written entries.

Some factors that may hinder legibility and put resident care at risk are:

- Poor handwriting,

- Use of unauthorized abbreviations,

- Felt tip pens,

- Improper corrections of errors, or

- Low toner or ink in computer printer cartridge.

Readable handwriting allows the interdisciplinary team to get the information they need to give care. Writing that is clear and legible allows staff to give the best care.

2.   Ink, Typewritten, Printed by Computer

All entries in the clinical record should be original documents and be written in permanent ink, typewritten or printed by a computer. It is best to use a medium point blue or black ballpoint pen. Colored ink, especially in fine point pens, can be difficult to read or photocopy. Some felt tip pens are not permanent and are erasable. In addition, entries made by felt tip pens may be illegible or may bleed through the paper making documentation on the reverse side of the page impossible to read.

When reports are printed by computer, a laser printer should be used. An inkjet printer is not permanent. The ink is water-soluble.

Pencil may not be used. Remember the example of writing a personal check. It would be unthinkable for a person to write a check in pencil. An erasure would easily change the amount of money specified. The same holds true for documentation of resident care.

3.   Dated

Each entry in the clinical record is dated. It is both unethical and illegal to pre-date or post-date an entry. Entries in the clinical record are identified with the date and time they are made. Documentation should be completed as soon as possible after an event or observation is made.

Always include the year when writing dates. A complete date including the year is essential to identify the time frame of each entry throughout the entire record. Many residents stay longer than one year and some for a number of years. Complete dates and even times may be needed to document a situation accurately.

Using only month and year for quarterly notes is <u>not</u> recommended. The resident's condition at the beginning of a month may be significantly different thirty days later. For example, a resident may suddenly have a change of condition during the month. If the entry did not include the day of the month, it might appear that the activity professional was unaware of the change in condition.

4.   Signature with Full Name and Title

Every entry in the clinical record must be validated with a signature. Again, consider the example of writing a personal check. If the check does not have a signature, the bank will not cash the check. If a credit card receipt does not have a signature, the amount due may not be honored.

The complete name and professional title of the person making the entry authenticates that entry. A health care professional must always write and sign their own entries. Never make an entry or sign an entry for someone else.

Information may be transcribed into the clinical record from a source completed by another health care professional. When doing so, identify the name and title of the person transcribing the information, and the name and title of the person who originally wrote the information.

For example, *Transcribed by Mary Jones, Activity Director, from Transfer Record (date) signed by Susan Smith, RN.*

Data entry by clerical staff into computer systems from handwritten worksheets is not considered transcription. The health care professional that completed the worksheet must review the computer printout and authenticate the information as correct with a complete signature.

For example, all Minimum Data Set (MDS) assessment information may be entered into the computer by medical record staff. The activity professional who completed the information for Section N of the MDS will sign the certification on the MDS Tracking Record to verify that the information in the MDS Section N is accurate.

From CMS Long Term Care RAI User's Manual

Nursing homes may use electronic signatures for clinical record documentation, including the MDS, when permitted to do so by state and local law and when authorized by the long term care facility policy. Facilities must have written policies in place to ensure proper security measures to protect the use of an electronic signature by anyone other than the person to which the electronic signature belongs.

---

5. Initials

Initials of the health care professional's name should not be used to authenticate narrative notes or assessments. Initials can be difficult to decipher and may cause problems with identifying the person who actually made an entry.

Federal regulations state that full signatures and titles are required on the Minimum Data Set (MDS) assessment. Initials may be used on flow sheets if the signature of the health care professional is also recorded somewhere on that same flow sheet.

6. Completing Forms

When completing forms or checklists, all questions and fields need to be answered. If the item is not applicable, mark the area as not applicable (*n/a*). Fields or questions left blank may lead to confusion. A reviewer does not know if the information was omitted or was not applicable (*n/a*).

7. Corrections

When there is an error in documentation, make a legal correction. Do not attempt to erase, write-over, block out or use whiteout. Strict rules apply to correcting clinical records. Improper corrections will invalidate the record for legal purposes. When records are unclear, they can affect resident care and become a liability.

For example, a personal check or credit card receipt with whiteout would not be valid. Likewise, a clinical record that has not been corrected properly would no longer be evidence of care.

PROCEDURE FOR LEGAL CORRECTION OF CLINICAL RECORD

To make a legal correction, follow these steps.

(a) Draw a single line through each word, phrase, or line of the material to be corrected. Make sure that the original information remains legible. Do not obliterate the information to be corrected.

(b) State that the information was an *error*, then write the date and initial the error message.

(c) Next record the correct information. The person making the correction then signs the entry with complete name and professional title.

If an entire page is in error and must be recopied, the original may not be discarded. The original page is marked as recopied, signed and dated by the person doing the transcription and filed with the corrected copy. The original entry made at the time the event occurred, along with the signature of the professional authenticating the notes, must always be available with the recopied material.

8.   Omissions in Documentation

At times it will be necessary to make an entry that is out of sequence or provide additional documentation to supplement or clarify entries previously written. These types of entries in the clinical record are identified as *Late Entry, Addendum or Clarification.*

Such entries may be used for assessments, orders, or narrative notes:

- *Late Entry* is documentation made when a pertinent or required entry was missed or not written in a timely manner. Late entries are made when documentation was not completed during the time period required, such as a late quarterly progress note.

- *Addendum* is used to provide additional information that was not included in the original chart entry. For example, information may be added to the chart about reasons that were later identified regarding why a resident did not participate in an activity.

- *Clarification* is written to add information to an original entry to avoid misinterpretation. Most often, clarifications are made to physician orders. For example, a physician may write an order that a resident may have a leave of absence for a weekend. The clarification may be necessary to indicate that the leave of absence is for the resident's birthday weekend at a daughter's home.

PROCEDURE FOR OMISSIONS IN DOCUMENTATION

The following steps are used to document out of sequence entries:

(a)   Identify the type of entry (*Late Entry, Addendum,* or *Clarification*) with current date and time.

(b)   Refer to the date and type of documentation (*Assessment, Orders, Progress Note*) that will be amended.

(c)   Complete the additional information and sign with name and title.

Examples: (Current Date) *Late entry for quarterly progress note*
(Due date that was missed)

(Current Date) *Addendum to Initial Assessment*
(Date of initial assessment)

(Current Date) *Clarification to Physician Order*
(Date of physician order)

Clinical documentation should always be done in a timely manner. Do not falsify the record by pre-dating or post-dating an entry.

Take care to make sure that chart entries are timely, complete and accurate. Frequent entries identified as *Late Entry* may raise questions about the accuracy of all the information contained in a clinical record.

9.   Chronological Order

The progress notes in the chart must be maintained in chronological order. Health care professionals expect to find information in predictable places in the clinical record. If reports are out of order, the information may not be found when needed. Incomplete information may lead to decisions that are not in the best interests of the resident.

Entries are recorded consecutively in the clinical record. <u>Do not</u> leave spaces or skip lines to allow someone else to document. When it is necessary to leave a blank section at the bottom of the progress notes and begin a new sheet of paper, line out that section of the progress note that is being left blank. The purpose of lining out the blank lines is to prevent someone from writing in the blank space. This is a protection for record integrity and will help keep the chart in chronological order.

10.   *Continued* Notes to Next Page

When a progress note is *continued* onto another page, write *continued* at the end of the page. This will show that the entry is completed on the next page. On the new page, indicate the date again, write *continued*, and record the remainder of the note. Conclude the documentation with a full signature.

By writing on both sheets that there is *continued* information on another page, those reviewing the notes are alerted that additional details of care are recorded elsewhere.

If continuations are not clearly identified, decisions could be made with incomplete information, increasing the risk of errors in treatment.

11.   Inappropriate Notes

Remember that the clinical record is the resident's record. Information contained in the record describes the resident's condition, problems, needs and treatment provided. Information regarding the facility's problems is not a part of the resident's treatment. Clinical record documentation reflects the professionalism of the person making the notes.

<u>Do not</u> write items in the record that are not related to the care of the resident. Complaints about other staff, blaming or criticizing others are not appropriate in the clinical record. The mechanism for correcting such complaints should be done by an administrative memorandum.

When writing narrative notes:

- Use specific language. Avoid vague or generalized statements.

- Do not speculate. State only the facts and objective information.

- Describe symptoms by manifestation or behavior.

- Use quotation marks for statements made by resident.

If it is necessary to refer to another resident to describe an event, the other resident's name should not be used. The clinical record should contain only documentation that pertains to the direct care of the resident.

C.   Maintaining the Clinical Record

Guidelines for maintaining a legal document need to be followed to assure the integrity of the clinical record. Records need to be stored in a manner to prevent loss of pages from the record and to prevent any damage or destruction from the physical elements. These guidelines apply to both paper and computerized records.

To be useful, the clinical record must be systematically organized. Reports must be clearly identified with the resident's name. Care should be taken to avoid misfiling reports. The purpose of the clinical record is to provide accurate, concise, and comprehensive health information about the resident.

1.   Unit Record

All resident health information must be centralized in the clinical record. Missing or late documentation may lead to unintentional errors by others who depend on the record for information. The health care professional must know all the facts to make decisions. Quality care is not possible if information is not timely, incomplete or inaccurate.

For example, if the activity professional is not informed that a resident is diabetic, snacks may be offered during a food-related activity that would not be appropriate for that resident. Although the activity professional has followed all regulations and standards of performance, a poor outcome may result for the resident. A diabetic resident may not be able to tolerate a snack that is too high in sugar or carbohydrate.

Complete and accurate information is the key to assuring quality care. Activity program assessments, care plans and progress notes must be completed on time. Positive outcomes can only be achieved if all health care professionals are working together, making decisions on reliable information. The clinical record is the source of resident health information for all members of the interdisciplinary team.

2.   Clinical Record Organization

The current record is usually maintained in a binder with section tabs for the various health care disciplines. Activity documentation will have its own tab divider. Be careful that all documentation is filed behind the correct divider. Misfiled reports can cause problems when health care professionals are not able to find the information needed.

If a resident stays for a long time and the chart becomes bulky, sections of the record may be thinned by medical record personnel. Such thinned records are usually maintained near the nursing station or in the medical record department. Initial activity assessments should remain in the chart as baseline documentation. However, progress notes and other flow sheets may be thinned out according to facility policy, such as after fifteen months or two years.

3.   Report Identification

Every page in the clinical record or computer screen must identify the resident by name, record number, and room location in the facility. This identification should be on both sides of every page whether handwritten or computer printed.

Resident identification information can be handwritten in ink, typewritten or printed by computer, stamped using an addressograph machine, or affixed by a label.

4.   Photocopies

The clinical record should contain original documents of reports completed by facility staff. Photocopied reports from other hospitals, laboratories, or outside providers may be included as part of the record.

Copies used as part of the clinical record must be permanent copies, such as from a photocopy or plain paper fax machine. Carbon copies, NCR (no carbon required) or thermal fax copies may fade or become illegible over time. Use these reports only on a temporary basis. If necessary, photocopy the temporary reports received on such paper. Retain the permanent photocopy in the clinical record. Discard the temporary fax copy in a confidential manner.

The availability of health information to others providing care for the resident is important to assure continuity and proper care. The clinical record may be duplicated so health information can be made available to other hospitals or health care providers. However, the original report always stays in the facility clinical record.

The clinical record must be written in a manner so that a legible photocopy or fax can be made. Intensely colored paper may not make a legible photocopy. Colored ink may be used, if the facility's photocopy equipment can clearly reproduce the record.

5. Facsimile (FAX) Copies

Fax copies are acceptable in the clinical record. A signature on the fax copy is valid according to federal laws. The original author does not have to countersign the fax copy when later visiting the facility. The original copy may be maintained at the originator's office to be produced upon request. Or the original may be sent to the nursing facility to be included in the clinical record and the fax copy may be discarded in a confidential manner.

Remember, thermal fax paper fades easily and is not a permanent record. Always photocopy a fax printed on a thermal paper machine to make a permanent document. Then use the photocopy in the clinical record or request that the sending party follow-up via mail with copies that are legible and permanent for use in the clinical record. The thermal fax copy may be discarded in a confidential manner once a permanent copy has been obtained. There is no problem with fax machines that print on regular paper.

D. Abbreviations

An approved abbreviation list should be maintained at the facility. This list is reviewed periodically to assure that the abbreviations used have been approved. Health care professionals who use abbreviations should ask for approval of all abbreviations that they intend to use. Approval is obtained from the committee that reviews resident care policies or quality assessment and assurance.

Use only facility-approved abbreviations. Studies have shown that some abbreviations contribute to medical errors. The Joint Commission on Accreditation of Hospitals and Organizations has identified *dangerous* abbreviations and acronyms and symbols. Your facility may also have a list of *Do not use* abbreviations.

COMMONLY USED ABBREVIATIONS

AD	Activity Director
ADL	activities of daily living
AKA	above the knee amputation
am	morning (before noon)
A&O	alert and oriented
BKA	below the knee amputation
c/o	complaint of
cont	continued
DOB	date of birth
Dx	diagnosis
ETOH	ethanol (alcohol)
Fx	fracture
HOH	hard of hearing
Hx	history of
IDT	interdisciplinary team
LOA	leave of absence
LN	licensed nurse
MD	medical doctor, physician
MDS	Minimum Data Set
neg	negative
NF	nursing facility
NKA	no known allergies
noc	night
NPO	nothing by mouth
NWB	non-weight bearing
OOB	out of bed
pm	afternoon/evening
prn	as needed
PTA	prior to admission
RAI	Resident Assessment Instrument
RAP	Resident Assessment Protocol
ROM	range of motion
SNF	skilled nursing facility
STAT	immediately
TPR	temperature, pulse & respiration
TTWB	touch toe weight bearing
Tx	treatment
w/c	wheelchair
WNL	within normal limits
wt	weight

Some examples of abbreviations found to be *error prone* are:

D/C	Discharge or discontinue
q.d. or QD	Once daily
OJ	Orange juice
TIW or tiw	3 times a week

Remember, if the person recording the information is the only one that knows what an abbreviation means, the information is useless. Others may not understand or may misinterpret unapproved abbreviations. The overuse of abbreviations also can produce documentation that is not informative or useful.

E.   Security of Protected Health Information

All or sections of clinical records, such as the resident assessment instrument and progress notes, may be completed by the use of computer-generated reports. Reports generated by computer software are processed and maintained in a manner to ensure the safety, integrity and confidentiality of the clinical record.

1.   Clinical Records

Protection of resident health information is an basic right for all residents. Both paper and computer information must be used in a manner that assures each resident the right to privacy. A federal law, known as the HIPAA Privacy and Security rules, govern how resident health information may be used and protected.

The clinical record is a legal document and must be stored in a manner to protect the record from loss, tampering or unauthorized access. This means that the clinical record should not be left unattended or in areas of public access. Do not leave clinical records open when not in use.

Records that identify residents by name should be stored in locked cabinets or in a locked office when not attended. Every health care professional has a duty to protect the security of resident health information.

The original clinical record or sections of the record may not be removed from the facility. If information for resident care is needed by other health care providers, such as when transferring the resident to the acute hospital, copies of necessary information can be provided.

Be alert that confidential health information may appear on documents that never become part of the clinical record. Some of these documents may be schedules of activities, flow sheets or memoranda. All resident health information must be protected from unlawful disclosure whether part of the legal clinical record or not.

Care must be taken to dispose of resident identified papers in a manner to protect the resident's privacy. Shredders are one recommended method. Be careful when recycling papers that resident names are protected from disclosure.

2. Facsimile (FAX)

If resident health information is faxed to other caregivers, procedures need to be followed to assure privacy of information.

- Use a fax cover sheet that identifies that the information being faxed is confidential. Provide a telephone number for the recipient to call back if the information is received in error.

- Be sure to confirm that the fax number is correct before sending the information. Use auto-dial for frequently used phone numbers to avoid misdialing errors.

- Fax machines should be located in a secure area away from public access.

3. Computers

Computers used for protected health information should be located in a secure area away from public access to protect privacy of information and prevent theft. A computer may be located at a nursing station that is off limits to residents and the public or in a private office with a locked door. Computer screens should be turned so that a passerby is unable to view the screen.

Use a personal identification code or password to access computer software. Passwords protect against unauthorized access to confidential resident health information. Passwords may be used only by the person to whom it is assigned. Passwords may not be shared with other personnel or consultants.

Once a user has logged on a computer program, the computer should not be left unattended. Security measures must be in place to prevent access or tampering by unauthorized users. Back up files on a regular basis to prevent loss of information.

4. E-Mail

Communicating with others about a resident's protected health information should be done with caution. HIPAA security rules require a facility to take steps to assure that e-mail is received only by the person entitled to the information. Encryption of the e-mail is not always possible, so there is risk that the information may end up in the wrong hands.

Use e-mail cautiously for communicating protected health information about a resident. At a minimum, include in the e-mail a confidentiality statement that warns the recipient that the information is confidential and if they have received this information in error that they must notify the sender.

An example of a confidentiality statement that can be included with either e-mail or fax of protected health information is:

This communication is intended solely for the addressee and is confidential. If you are not the intended recipient, any disclosure, copying, distribution or any action taken or omitted to be taken in reliance on it, is prohibited and may be unlawful.

(For Faxes) If you have received this communication in error, please notify me immediately by telephone for instructions to destroy this fax in a confidential manner..

(For E-Mail) If you have received this communication in error, please notify me immediately by replying to this message and deleting it from your computer.

Selecting Forms

KEY POINTS AND SUMMARY OF CHAPTER

Activity program documentation is written on three basic kinds of forms: Assessments, Flow Sheets and Progress Notes.

The Minimum Data Set (MDS) and a supplemental assessment form will contain the information needed to assess a resident's activity needs.

Flow Sheet charting saves time in documenting care and finding needed information.

Follow guidelines for forms design to assure appropriate style and use.

A.   Assessment Forms

Nursing facilities participating in the Medicare and Medicaid program are required to use the Resident Assessment Instrument (RAI) that includes the Minimum Data Set (MDS) and Resident Assessment Protocols (RAPs). The MDS Section N addresses activity pursuit patterns. However, the MDS Section N does not contain all of the information the activity director needs to identify resident needs and strengths and develop an appropriate and individualized plan of care.

The Resident Assessment Instrument (RAI) system uses the MDS data to trigger Resident Assessment Protocols (RAPs). The RAPs contain guidelines for an in-depth assessment of the resident. This further information regarding the resident needs is documented as a supplemental assessment in the clinical record based on the RAP guidelines.

Choosing and/or designing an appropriate form will may documentation easier and prevent charting errors. Well designed forms will allow efficient communication with the interdisciplinary team.

1.   **Types of Assessment Forms**

Assessment forms used by activity professionals include:

•   Minimum Data Set (MDS) Section N Activity Pursuit Patterns

•   Activity needs assessment form (Supplemental RAP assessment)

Supplemental assessment forms are used to collect additional information about the resident's needs, strengths, preferences and any issues identified in the Resident Assessment Protocols (RAPs).

When selecting a supplemental assessment form, the content should include enough information to demonstrate that the RAPs have been used in the development of the activity plan.

Activity Needs Assessment should address:

Physical limitations
Functional status
Mental acuity
Social skills
Psychological well-being
Recreational preferences
Spiritual needs
Cultural values
Customary routines.

---

2.   **Selecting Forms**

The selection of supplemental assessment forms is based on writing style and individual preference. Paragraph style forms are suitable for narrative charting. Interventions such as activity attendance patterns are usually documented on flow sheets.

Supplemental assessments may be written

•   in a narrative format on the activity progress notes, or

•   on a structured form that contains an outline of required information.

If a structured form is selected, it may simply provide an outline of topics to be assessed or it may be structured as a check off system.

SAMPLE NURSING FACILITY

ACTIVITY PROGRAM ASSESSMENT
Page One

Diagnosis_____ Birth date_____

Precautions: Allergies_____   Nutrition_____
                        Mobility_____   Other_____

Customary Routines: _____
                        _____

Physical Deficits: Hearing_____
                        Vision_____
                        Dexterity_____
                        Communication_____
                        Other_____

Functional Status: Ambulatory (Self)_____
                        Assisted Ambulation_____
                        Wheelchair_____
                        Bedfast_____
                        Other_____

Mental Acuity: Alert_____
                        Oriented_____
                        Confused_____
                        Lethargic_____
                        Other_____

Social Interactions: Family_____
                        Visitors_____
                        Prefers Groups_____
                        Prefers Alone_____
                        Other_____

Psychological: Behavior_____
                        Motivation_____
                        Other_____

Religion_____   Cultural Needs_____

Language_____   Holidays_____

RESIDENT NO_____ RESIDENT NAME_____ROOM NO____

ACTIVITY PROGRAM ASSESSMENT
Page Two

Recreational Preferences:

Art/Crafts	☐	Movies	☐
Bingo	☐	Music	☐
Cards	☐	Needlework	☐
Collecting	☐	Outdoors	☐
Contests	☐	Pets	☐
Cooking	☐	Sports	☐
Family	☐	Television	☐
Flower Arranging	☐	Woodworking	☐
Games	☐	Word Games	☐
Gardening	☐	Writing	☐
Group Exercises	☐	Other_____	☐

LONG TERM GOALS:_____

_____

SHORT TERM GOALS:

Increase social interactions	☐
Improve morale and sense of well-being	☐
Increase physical stamina and tolerance	☐
Increase attention span	☐
Reality orientation	☐
Stimulate imagination and decision making	☐
Develop social network and support group	☐
Sensory stimulation	☐
Other_____	☐

Plan: Group Activities:_____

_____

        Independent Activities:_____

_____

        Family Involvement:_____

_____

DATE_____SIGNED BY_____A.D.

RESIDENT NO_____ RESIDENT NAME_____ROOM NO____

SAMPLE NURSING FACILITY
ACTIVITY PROGRAM ASSESSMENT
Page One

Diagnosis_____Birth date_____

Precautions:

Customary Routines:

Physical Deficits:

Functional Status:

Mental Acuity:

Social Interactions:

Psychological:

Religion_____   Cultural Needs_____

Language_____   Holidays_____

RESIDENT NO___ RESIDENT NAME_____ RM NO_____

ACTIVITY PROGRAM ASSESSMENT
Page Two

Recreational Preferences:

LONG TERM GOALS:

SHORT TERM GOALS:

Plan: Group Activities:

             Independent Activities:

             Family Involvement:

DATE_____SIGNED BY_____A.D.

RESIDENT NO____ RESIDENT NAME_____ RM NO_____

B. Flow Sheets

Flow sheet charting is a useful method of recording information about the resident in a timesaving manner. It also provides a quick method for review of information. Information is easily compared and trends spotted.

Flow Sheets save time in recording and finding information. They are useful to document attendance records and one to one room visits.

For example, an activity attendance record is usually a flow sheet that can be reviewed quickly to identify the resident's activity attendance pattern. This information cannot be easily found if recorded in progress notes. Months of narrative progress notes would need to be read in a time consuming effort to determine if the resident had changes in activity levels.

Flow sheet charting can also be considered a type of narrative charting. If the flow sheet is designed so entries are made according to a key that is printed on the form, it is considered narrative charting. Checkmark entries are not considered narrative charting.

A combination form that includes a flow sheet and a progress notes in one form can also be useful. The flow sheet can be used to document the resident's activity for a quarter. Then, at the end of the quarter, the activity director can review the resident's activity attendance and reactions. An activity progress note is written to summarize and evaluate the resident's response and participation in activity programs.

Flow sheets provide a comparative display of information for easy retrieval and evaluation. Flow sheet charting is useful for recording activity program participation simply and quickly.

C. Progress Notes

Progress notes are narrative evaluations of the resident's response to the plan of care and the progress, maintenance or regress in respect to the goals identified in the care plan. The notes are written at the end of each quarter based on information gathered on flow sheets and from direct observation of the resident.

Usually, a plain lined form is suitable for progress notes. However, consider a form that combines a flow sheet with the progress notes. The one to one visit flow sheet and group activity attendance flow sheet can be combined on one side of the page. The progress note can be printed on the opposite side of the page. When the quarter has ended, the activity director simply reviews and compares the flow sheet data and writes a progress note. Once this is completed the form is placed in the clinical record.

SAMPLE NURSING FACILITY

ACTIVITY ATTENDANCE RECORD
Page One

Month of_____ Year_____

ACTIVITY	1	2	3	4	5	6	7	8	9	10	11	12	13	14	15	16	17	18	19	20	21	22	23	24	25	26	27	28	29	30	31
Group:																															
In Room:																															
One to One:																															

Month of_____ Year_____

ACTIVITY	1	2	3	4	5	6	7	8	9	10	11	12	13	14	15	16	17	18	19	20	21	22	23	24	25	26	27	28	29	30	31
Group:																															
In Room:																															
One to One:																															

Participation Key: A = Active; P = Passive; R = Refused

RESIDENT NO___ RESIDENT NAME_____ RM NO_____

ACTIVITY ATTENDANCE RECORD
Page Two

Month of_____ Year_____

ACTIVITY	1	2	3	4	5	6	7	8	9	10	11	12	13	14	15	16	17	18	19	20	21	22	23	24	25	26	27	28	29	30	31
Group:																															
In Room:																															
One to One:																															

ACTIVITY PROGRESS NOTE

Problems/Needs:_____

_____

_____

Goals/Objectives:_____

_____

_____

Response to Activity Plan:_____

_____

_____

_____

DATE_____SIGNED BY_____A.D.

RESIDENT NO___ RESIDENT NAME_____ RM NO_____

SAMPLE NURSING FACILITY

ACTIVITY ATTENDANCE RECORD
Page One

Month of_____ Year_____

1	2	3	4	5	6	7	8	9	10	11	12	13	14	15	16	17	18	19	20	21	22	23	24	25	26	27	28	29	30	31

Month of_____ Year_____

1	2	3	4	5	6	7	8	9	10	11	12	13	14	15	16	17	18	19	20	21	22	23	24	25	26	27	28	29	30	31

Month of_____ Year_____

1	2	3	4	5	6	7	8	9	10	11	12	13	14	15	16	17	18	19	20	21	22	23	24	25	26	27	28	29	30	31

ATTENDANCE KEY

Group:

Arts/Crafts	A	Movies	L	Room Visits:	
Bingo	B	Music	M	Books	1
Cards	C	Needlework	N	Crafts	2
Contests	D	Outdoors	O	Discussion	3
Cooking	K	Pets	P	Exercises	4
Exercises	E	Sports	S	Games	5
Flowers	F	Television	T	Music	6
Games	G	Word Games	U	Sensory Stimulation	7
Gardening	H	Writing	W	Volunteer	8
				Family	9

RESIDENT NO___ RESIDENT NAME_____ RM NO_____

SAMPLE NURSING FACILITY

ACTIVITY PROGRESS NOTES
Page Two

Problems/Needs:_____

_____

_____

Goals/Objectives:_____

_____

_____

Response to Activity Plan:_____

_____

_____

_____

_____

_____

_____

_____

_____

_____

_____

_____

DATE_____SIGNED BY_____A.D.

RESIDENT NO___ RESIDENT NAME_____RM NO_____

Progress notes should to be filed in the clinical record in chronological order. This may be latest on top or in strict date order. If using the backside of a progress note for recording, strict date order works best. Keeping chart forms in the proper sequence will avoid confusion. If latest on top filing in the current record is used, three holes can be punched on both the right and left margins. When the backside of the form is used, it simply can be turned over.

D.   Forms Design

Whether designing a form or selecting a preprinted form, there are guidelines that will help in the selection process. Poorly designed forms can lead to charting errors. Be aware that unnecessary forms cause unnecessary paperwork. Whenever possible, avoid duplicating any information that is already included on another form in the clinical record.

For example, information collected in the MDS does not have to be repeated on other forms. If there is reason to make duplicate entries of information, be sure all areas agree and are not in conflict.

DESIGN GUIDELINES

(a)   Allow ¼ inch space at top of form

(b)   Name of facility should appear on form

(c)   The form must have a title

(d)   For binder systems, the left-hand margin must have ¾ inch allowance for hole punch

(e)   Content of the forms must include a place for a date and a signature

(h)   Space must be provided for at least the resident name, number and room.

A pilot or testing period with a small supply of a new form is recommended. Errors and revisions are quickly spotted and can be corrected without undue expense. Corrected versions of the form are then available on a timely basis.

To avoid confusion when working with forms revision, it is helpful to include a form number and date of current revision of the form. Often multiple versions of a form circulate throughout the facility, making it difficult to determine which is the current form.

When creating a new form, it is good practice to justify the need for the form by using the following criteria:

a.   Identify the Need:
         What purpose?
         Why the change?
         Where will it be used, filed or stored?
         What present form does it replace?
             Present number on hand (inventory)?
         If not replacing another form,
             how was the information collected previously?
             how will the new form improve the record?

b.   Evaluate the Use:
         Who will use?
         Procedures for completing form?
         Typed or handwritten? Computer generated?
         Estimated annual quantity?
         Compatibility and interface with other forms?

Resident Rights

KEY POINTS AND SUMMARY OF CHAPTER

The activity program is an essential part of the quality of life for residents in a nursing facility.

Activity programs are designed to promote resident dignity, enhance self-esteem and self-worth and allow opportunities for choice and self-determination, and accommodation of the resident's special needs.

The activity professional has an obligation to maintain the confidentiality of medical or personal information about residents.

A.   Resident Rights

Resident rights are the hallmark of the federal regulations governing nursing facilities. Each resident has the right to be provided care in a manner and in an environment that treats each resident as a person, recognizes each resident's individual needs and enhances each resident's quality of life.

Quality of life depends on:

- each resident being treated with dignity and respect,

- recognition of each resident's individuality,

- allowing the resident to make choices about his or her life in the facility, and

- accommodating the resident's special needs.

B.   Quality of Life

The activity program is an essential part of assuring the quality of life in the nursing facility. A well-developed activity plan with appropriate activities that are chosen based on the resident's needs, strengths, and preferences:

- maintains the resident's dignity,

- allows self-determination and accommodation of unique needs,

- enhances self-worth,

- promotes motivation and sense of well-being, and

- assists in achieving positive outcomes of care.

Quality of life is obvious through observation. Look around, see what residents are doing. Listen to the tone of conversations between staff and residents. By looking and listening it is easy to determine if staff are assuring resident rights.

Very simply, staff actions demonstrate that resident rights are respected, such as:

- Residents are well groomed and appropriately dressed.

- Staff talks and listens to residents, providing explanations to the resident when care is given.

- Residents are informed of activities that are appropriate to the resident.

- Activity programs take place according to the posted activity calendar.

- Residents are not sitting in hallways with no apparent purpose or involvement in facility daily life.

- Staff handles behavior of the residents, such as crying out, disrobing, agitation, rocking, or pacing by residents.

Section 483.15 titled *Quality of Life* contains regulations and interpretive guidelines which are instructions to surveyors on how to determine if the activity program is in compliance. The intent of these regulations is to create and sustain an environment that humanizes and individualizes the resident. The interpretive guidelines give instructions and examples for surveyors to determine if staff interactions provide residents with a sense of dignity.

CFR Section 483.15 Quality of Life

§483.15 A facility must care for its residents in a manner and in an environment that promotes maintenance or enhancement of each resident's quality of life.

(a)   *Dignity.*

      The facility must promote care for residents in a manner and in an environment that maintains or enhances each resident's dignity and respect in full recognition of his or her individuality.

(b)   *Self-determination and participation.*

      The resident has the right to--

      (1)   *Choose activities, schedules and health care consistent with his or her interests, assessments and plans of care;*

      (2)   *Interact with members of the community both inside and outside the facility; and*

      (3)   *Make choices about aspects of his or her life in the facility that are significant to the resident.*

(d)   *Participation in other activities. . .*

      A resident has the right to participate in social, religious, and community activities that do not interfere with the rights of other residents in the facility.

(e)   *Accommodation of needs. A resident has the right to --*

      (1)   *Reside and receive services in the facility with reasonable accommodation of individual needs and preferences, except when the health or safety of the individual or other residents would be endangered; and*

      (2)   *Receive notice before the resident's room or roommate in the facility is changed.*

Interpretive Guidelines §483.15 (a) Dignity.

Dignity means that in their interactions with residents, staff carries out activities that assist the resident to maintain and enhance his/her self-esteem and self-worth.

For example:

- *Grooming residents as they wish to be groomed (e.g., hair combed and styled, beards shaved/trimmed, nails clean and clipped);*

- *Assisting residents to dress in their own clothes appropriate to the time of day and individual preferences;*

- *Assisting residents to attend activities of their own choosing;*

- *Respecting resident's private space and property, e.g., not changing radio or television station without resident's permission;*

- *Knocking on doors and requesting permission to enter, closing doors as requested by the resident;*

- *Not moving or inspecting resident's personal possessions without permission;*

- *Respecting resident's social status, speaking respectfully, listening carefully, treating resident with respect (e.g., addressing the resident with a name of the resident's choice, not excluding residents from conversations or discussing residents in community setting; and*

- *Focusing on residents as individuals when they talk to them and addressing residents as individuals when providing care and services.*

Procedures §483.15 (a) Dignity.

Throughout the survey, observe:

Do staff show respect for residents? When staff interact with a resident, do staff pay attention to the resident as an individual? Do staff respond in a timely manner to the resident's requests for assistance? In group activities, do staff focus attention on the group of residents? Or, do staff appear distracted when they interact with residents? For example, do staff continue to talk with each other while doing a task for a resident(s) as if she/he were not present?

1.   Dignity

Surveyors are instructed to observe the activity levels of residents to evaluate if residents are being treated with courtesy and respect. Dignity is observable. The manner in which staff address residents reflects dignity. Labels such as *the screamer*, *the complainer* and pet names such as *Gramps, honey, sweetie* are demeaning and inappropriate.

Staff should focus on the resident as an individual when talking and explain the care and/or services being provided. have conversations in the presence of a resident that excludes his or her participation. Be careful about talking about a resident in settings within the facility where others can overhear.

2.   Self-determination

The activity program enhances the resident's quality of life when it includes opportunities for choice and self-determination. Whenever possible, the activity plan should allow the resident to work with the staff to set up daily schedules that consider the resident's former life style, customary routines and personal choices. Voicing opinions, participating in resident council, making suggestions are considered empowerment activities.

Interpretive Guidelines §483.15 (b) Self-determination and Participation.

The intent of this requirement is to specify that the facility must create an environment that is respectful of the right of each resident to exercise his or her autonomy regarding what the resident considers to be important facets of his or her life.

> *For example, if a facility changes its policy and prohibits smoking, it must allow current residents who smoke to continue smoking in an area that maintains the quality of life for these residents. Weather permitting, this may be an outside area. Residents admitted after the facility changes its policy must be informed of this policy at admission.*

Or, if a resident mentions that her therapy is scheduled at the time of her favorite television program, the facility should accommodate the resident to the extent that it can.

Procedures §483.15 (b) Self-determination and Participation.

Observe how well staff know each resident and what aspects of life are important to him/her. Determine if staff make adjustments to allow residents to exercise choice and self-determination.

The right of self-determination is intended to create a home-like environment that allows that residents to plan their daily schedules and making choices, if able. Activity staff can create and accommodate residents special needs.

- Offer residents choices of activity programs to attend.

- If a resident refuses to attend group activities, offer one-to-one interventions and in room activities.

- If a resident has a complaint, help the resident to resolve it.

- Consider and accommodate the resident's customary routines in the resident's activity participation.

- Obtain resident and family input regarding activity choices.

- Come to know each resident and what aspects of life are important to him or her.

There is a fine line between helping a resident and taking away opportunities to make choices. Allow residents to make choices at the level of their abilities. Let the residents decide how they spend their time, both inside and outside the facility.

3.   Accommodation of Needs

Many residents in nursing homes require certain accommodation to meet their unique needs. Staff may need to make adjustments to allow residents to exercise choice and self-determination.

For example, accommodation of needs can be necessary for leisure activity choices, food preferences, telephone access, protection of personal property, and special accommodations for married couples.

Familiar objects and routines can provide residents with a sense of comfort and make the nursing facility feel more home-like rather than an institution. This can reduce some of the sense of loss and promote individuality. Activity staff can develop plans to accommodate a resident's needs and choices for how he/she spends time, both inside and outside the facility.

Married couples both of whom reside in the facility have the right to decide if they share the same room. A spouse who resides in the community may request privacy during visits.

Accommodation of needs may require adaptations of environment or planned staff interventions.

Interpretive Guidelines §483.15 (e) Accommodation of Needs

Reasonable accommodation of individual needs and preference is defined as the facility's efforts to individualize the resident's environment.

The facility's physical environment and staff behaviors should be conducive to assisting the resident's maintenance and/or achievement of independent function, dignity, and well-being. The resident's own preferences and staff assessment and care plans are used to develop appropriate interventions to assure accommodation of the resident's need. The facility should attempt to adapt such things as schedules, call systems, and room arrangements to accommodate resident's preferences, desires and unique needs.

Procedures §483.15 (e) Accommodation of Needs

Observe resident-staff interaction and determine to what extent staff attempt to accommodate residents' preferences. . .

- *Does the facility respond to resident's stated needs and preferences?*

- *How have resident's needs been accommodated?*

- *Do environmental adaptations enhance resident's independence, self-control and highest practicable well-being?*

- *Is the fit between residents' needs and environment positive?*

- *If the resident is unable to express needs and preferences that would individualize care, has the family expressed the resident's routine and has the facility responded?*

Review the extent to which the facility adapts the physical environment to enable residents to maintain unassisted functioning. These adaptations include, but are not limited to:

1. *Furniture and adaptive equipment that enables residents to participate in resident preferred activities.*

2. *Measures that:*
    a. *Enable residents with dementia to walk freely;*
    b. *Reorient and remotivate residents with restorative potential (e.g., displaying easily readable calendars and clocks, wall hanging evocative of the lives of residents*

> c. *Promote conversation and socialization (pictures and decorations that speak to the resident's age cohort).*
>
> *Determine if staff use appropriate measures to facilitate communication with residents who have difficulty communicating. For example, if necessary, does staff get at eye level, or remove a resident from noisy surroundings.*
>
> *Determine if staff communicate effectively with residents with cognitive impairments, such as referring in a non-contradictory way to what residents are saying, and addressing what residents are trying to express to the agenda behind their behavior.*

C.   Refusal

The resident's right to choice may result in resident or family refusal of activities or treatments. Offer explanations as to the rationale and importance of treatments and services but do not force residents to accept care.

Steps to take when a resident refuses care:

- treat with kindness, offer alternatives,

- counsel resident regarding necessity of treatment,

- report refusal to supervisor, and

- document refusal in health record.

Offer choices whenever possible:

- activities to attend,

- selection of clothing to wear,

- food preferences (likes or dislikes), or

- support comfort measures for end-of-life.

Refusal by a resident can mean many things. It is important to take time to determine why a resident does not want to participate in activity programs. Decreased participation is a trigger in the RAI-MDS process. The activity professional should consider various underlying causes. Do the available activities correspond to the residents lifetime values, attitudes and expectations? Does the resident consider activities a waste of time? Have activities requiring a lower energy level been considered such as reading a book or talking with friends?

CFR Section 483.10(b)(4) Right to Refuse Treatment

§483.10(b)(4) The resident has the right to refuse treatment. . .

Interpretive Guidelines §483.10(b)(4) Right to Refuse Treatment

The facility should determine exactly what the resident is refusing and why. To the extent the facility is able, it should address the resident's concern. . . The facility is expected to assess the reasons for this resident's refusal, clarify and educate the resident as to the consequences of refusal, offer alternative treatments, and continue to provide all other services.

If a resident's refusal of treatment brings about a significant change, the facility should reassess the resident and institute care planning changes. A resident's refusal of treatment does not absolve a facility from providing a resident with care that allows him/her to maintain his/her highest practicable physical, mental and psycho-social well-being in the context of making that refusal.

Observe resident-staff interaction and determine to what extent staff attempt to accommodate residents' preferences. . . Determine what happens when a resident states a preference in the form of a refusal. How does the staff attempt to learn what the resident is refusing and why, and make adjustments to an extent practicable to meet the resident's needs?

D. Privacy

1. Personal Privacy

Resident rights provide that a resident can expect personal privacy during care and treatment. Examinations and treatments are never performed in public areas of the building. Only authorized staff directly involved in treatment should be present when treatments are given. Those not involved in the care of the individual should not be present without the resident's consent while he/she is receiving personal care or treatment.

Be aware of residents' appearance when attending activities or whenever they are in any public area of the facility. Are they dressed properly with clothing buttoned and correctly fastened. Are they sitting in a dignified manner to avoid any improper exposure? For example, use lap robes if residents are unable to sit in a modest position.

---

2.   Confidentiality of Protected Health Information

Health care professionals are entrusted with personal health information regarding residents. This incurs an obligation and trust to maintain the confidentiality of all medical and personal information about residents. Those not involved in the care of the resident may not have access to a resident's health information unless specifically authorized by the resident or the resident's responsible person.

The Health Insurance Portability and Accountability Act (HIPAA) includes the Privacy Rule that applies to all providers of health care. These national standards protect a resident's clinical records and other personal health information.

The HIPAA Privacy Rule requires the facility to:

- Notify residents about their privacy rights and how their information can be used.

- Adopt and implement privacy procedure.

- Train employees so that they understand the privacy procedures.

- Designate a privacy officer and a security officer.

- Secure clinical records, whether in paper form or in a computer, so that they are not readily available to those who do not need them.

Personal and clinical records include all types of records the facility might keep on a resident, whether they are medical, social, fund accounts, automated, computerized or other.

Do not discuss residents:

- outside of the facility (on bus going home).

- where visitors or other residents can overhear.

Resident care may be discussed:

- at interdisciplinary team conferences.

- with other health professionals.

Always be aware to whom you are speaking. Do you know that this is a person who is authorized to receive protected health information? Be aware of where you are speaking. Can those not involved in resident care overhear what you are saying?

CFR Section 483.10(e) Privacy

§483.10(e)   Privacy

The resident has the right to personal privacy and confidentiality of his or her personal and clinical records.

> *(1)   Personal privacy includes accommodations, medical treatment, written and telephone communications, personal care, visits, and meetings of family and resident groups, but this does not require the facility to provide a private room for each resident;*

> *(2)   ...The resident may approve or refuse the release of personal and clinical records to any individual outside the facility.*

> *(3)   The resident's right to refuse release of personal and clinical records does not apply when --*

> > *(i)   The resident is transferred to another health care institution, or*
> > *(ii)   Record release is required by law.*

Interpretive Guidelines §483.10(e) Privacy

Right to privacy means the resident has the right to privacy with whomever the resident wishes. Privacy should include full visual, and, to the extent desired, for visits or other activities, auditory privacy. Private space may be created flexibly and need not be dedicated solely for visitation purposes.

For example, privacy for visitation or meetings might be arranged by using a dining area between meals, a vacant chapel, office or room; or an activities area when activities are not in progress. Arrangements for private space could be accomplished through cooperation between the facility's administration and resident or family groups so that private space is provided for those requesting it without infringement on the rights of other residents.

Questions from family and friends may be answered in a general manner regarding their condition depending on their involvement with care. Questions about detailed medical treatment should be referred to the doctor or charge nurse. Such questions are answered on a need to know basis, respecting the resident's right to privacy.

Hospital elevators, hallways and cafeterias are frequently places where staff may have conversations regarding confidential information that could be overheard. <u>Do not</u> discuss medical histories within earshot of strangers.

Actions that assure resident confidentiality and privacy:

- Knock on door when entering a resident's room.

- Do not leave charts open or flow sheets posted in public view.

- Do not open or read resident's mail unless requested.

Confidentiality <u>does not</u> prohibit sharing resident information among members of the health care team. To give the best possible care to the resident, all members of the health care team must be informed of the resident's condition and plan of care. Sharing information at change of shift report or at care plan conferences is not a violation of confidentiality. However, change of shift reporting and care plan conferences should be conducted in an area where other residents and visitors cannot overhear the discussion. Be aware of indiscreet conversation in public areas of the facility

Federal Regulations

> ### KEY POINTS AND SUMMARY OF CHAPTER
>
> The regulations for activity programs are found in the section of the regulations titled *Quality of Life.*
>
> The facility must provide for an ongoing program of activities designed to meet, in accordance with the comprehensive assessment, the interests and the physical, mental and psychosocial well-being of each resident.
>
> Facilities are surveyed on an annual basis by state inspectors. Surveyors will observe activities, interview residents and families and review clinical records to determine substantial compliance with regulations.

Nursing facilities participating in the Medicare and/or Medicaid programs must follow federal regulations for skilled nursing facilities. In addition, States have their own regulations. The complete text of the federal regulations developed by the Centers for Medicare and Medicaid Services (CMS) for skilled nursing facilities can be found in Section 42, Code of Federal Regulations, Part 483, et al.

In 2004 CMS converted its manuals containing regulations and guidance to surveyors from paper-based to web-based manuals. The regulations and interpretive guidelines are found on the CMS website for their program manuals (http://www.cms.hhs.gov/manuals). The manual that addresses skilled nursing facilities regulations is the State Operations Manual (Pub 100-7). The regulations and guidelines are found in Appendix PP.

In this chapter the text of the federal regulations for the activity program is provided as well as CMS's instructions to surveyors on how to evaluate the facility's compliance with the regulations. The guidance to surveyors is not regulation but is used to assist surveyors to determine if the facility has met the regulations.

A. Activity Program

The primary goal of the activity program is to enhance the quality of the resident's life and assist the resident to achieve his or her maximum functional potential. Activity planning is a universal need for all residents.

The activity program is integrated with the comprehensive assessment and inter-disciplinary care plan. The activity plan for each individual resident should complement the plans of other healthcare disciplines. Frequently activities can supplement interventions developed by other disciplines, such as exercise programs, passing nourishments and reality orientation.

CFR Section 483.15(f)(1) Activities

§483.15(f)(1) Activities.

(1)   The facility must provide for an ongoing program of activities designed to meet, in accordance with the comprehensive assessment, the interests and the physical, mental and psychosocial well-being of each resident.

(2)   The activities program must be directed by a qualified professional who

(i)   Is a qualified therapeutic recreation specialist or an activities professional who--

(A)   Is licensed or registered, if applicable, by the State in which practicing;

(B)   Is eligible for certification as a therapeutic recreation specialist or as an activities professional by a recognized accrediting body on or after October 1, 1990; or

(ii)   Has 2 years of experience in a social or recreational program within the last 5 years, 1 of which was full-time in a patient activities program in a health care setting; or

(iii)   Is a qualified occupational therapist or occupational therapy assistant; or

(iv)   Has completed a training course approved by the State.

Interpretive Guidelines §483.15(f)(1) Activities.

Because the activities program should occur within the context of each resident's comprehensive assessment and care plan, it should be multi-faceted and reflect each individual resident's needs. Therefore, the activity program should provide stimulation or solace; promote physical, cognitive and/or emotional health; enhance, to the extent practicable, each resident's physical and mental status; and promote each resident's self-respect by providing, for example, activities that support self-expression and choice.

Activities can occur at anytime and are not limited to formal activities being provided by the activity staff. Others involved may be any facility staff, volunteers and visitors.

An activity plan is developed to encourage residents toward restoration of self-care and the resumption of normal activities. Activities may include hobbies or interests pursued independently by the resident, such as reading the newspaper or watching sports on television. For those who cannot realistically resume normal activities, interventions are developed to prevent further mental or physical deterioration. Activity interventions for end-of-life may include comfort measures to provide solace, spirituality, and non-drug interventions to relieve pain.

B. Survey Process

Facilities are surveyed on an annual basis by state inspectors. The purpose of the survey is to determine if the facility is in substantial compliance with federal regulations. A review of the activity program is part of the survey process.

During the standard survey process, surveyors will observe activities, interview residents and families and review clinical records to determine:

• Compliance with residents' rights and quality of life requirements.

• The accuracy of the residents' comprehensive assessments and the adequacy of care plans based on these assessments

• The quality of services furnished, as measured by quality indicators of medical, nursing, rehabilitation care and drug therapy, dietary and nutrition services, *activities* and social participation, sanitation and infection control; and

- The effectiveness of the physical environment to empower residents, accommodate resident needs, and maintain resident safety.

The standard survey process is made up of seven (7) tasks:

Task 1:   Off-site Survey Preparation

Task 2 :   A.   Entrance Conference
             B.   On Site Preparatory Activities

Task 3   Initial Tour

Task 4:   Sample Selection

Task 5:   Information Gathering
             General Observations of the Facility
             Kitchen/Food Service Observation
             Resident Review
             Quality of Life Assessment
             Medication Pass
             Quality Assessment and Assurance Review
             Abuse Prohibition Review

Task 6:   Information Analysis for Deficiency Determination

Task 7:   Exit Conference

Survey protocols are used by surveyors to measure compliance with federal regulations. The protocols developed for surveyors by CMS are the authorized interpretations of mandatory regulations or requirements.

Prior to visiting a facility for survey, off site survey preparations are completed. Surveyors review information from the State MDS database to determine the facility's unique characteristics, such as, a high prevalence of young or male residents or residents with psychiatric diagnosis. From the MDS information reported, surveyors will identify concerns about the activities program meeting cultural needs, interests, preferences and the number of residents who have little or no meaningful activity involvement.

When the surveyors arrive, an entrance conference is held with administrative staff. The survey team will request certain information they need, including a copy of the activity calendar. Also the surveyors post signs announcing that a survey is being performed and that the surveyors are available to meet in private with residents or family who

---

have concerns. These signs are placed in areas that are easily observable by residents and visitors.

As soon as the entrance conference has been completed, surveyors will take an initial tour of the facility. During the initial tour and throughout the survey, the surveyors are instructed to observe individual, group and bedside activities to assess the quality of the activity program. Staff may be asked to identify those residents who have no family or significant others. The purpose is to determine if the activity program meets the interests, preferences and needs of the residents.

Probes §483.15(f)(1) Activities

Observe individual, group and bedside activities.

1. *Are residents who are confined or choose to remain in their rooms provided with in-room activities in keeping with life-long interest (e.g., music, reading, visits with individuals who share their interests or reasonable attempts to connect the resident with such individuals) and in-room projects they can work on independently? Do any facility staff members assist the resident with activities he or she can pursue independently?*

2. *If residents sit for long period of time with no apparently meaningful activities, is the cause:*

   a. *Resident choice;*

   b. *Failure of any staff or volunteers either to inform residents when activities are occurring or to encourage resident involvement in activities;*

   c. *Lack of assistance with ambulation;*

   d. *Lack of sufficient supplies and/or staff to facilitate attendance and participation in the activity programs.*

   e. *Program design that fails to reflect the interests or ability levels of residents, such as activities that are too complex?*

Based on observations during the initial tour and review of the facility characteristics reported on the MDS, the surveyors will select a sample of residents to review. Evaluation will include observation, interview and clinical record review.

Some additional factors that will be considered for the sample selection will be:

- New admissions, especially if admitted during the previous 14 days. Even though the Resident Assessment Instrument (RAI) is not required to be completed for these residents, the facility must plan care from the first day of each resident's admission;

- Residents most at risk of neglect and abuse, i.e., residents who have dementia; no or infrequent visitors, psychosocial, interactive, and/or behavioral dysfunction; or residents who are bedfast and totally dependent on care;

- Residents receiving hospice services;

- Residents with end-stage renal disease;

- Residents under the age of 55;

- Residents with mental illness or mental retardation; and

- Residents who communicate with non-oral communication devices, sign language, or who speak a language other than the dominate language of the facility.

During information gathering, the surveyors will review clinical records, observe the activity programs, both as scheduled and those activities pursued independently by residents. Residents and families will be interviewed and asked questions regarding the care that is provided.

C. Activity Calendar

During the entrance conference the surveyors will ask to review the activity calendars for the last three months. This information must be made available within one hour of the request.

The review of the activity calendar will determine if the formal activity program:

- reflects schedules, choices and rights of the residents,

- offers activities at hours convenient to the residents (e.g., morning, afternoon, some evenings and weekends),

- reflects the cultural and religious interests of the resident population, and

- would appeal to both men and women and all age groups living in facility.

Even though surveyors are instructed to ask for the activity calendar, the survey instructions note that federal regulations do not require that an activity calendar be maintained. Local and state regulations, however, may require an activity calendar. Be sure to check local and state regulations for exact requirements. If there are no requirements and no activity calendar is maintained, inform the surveyors that a calendar is not maintained.

D. Resident Interviews

A sample of residents and family members will be interviewed. The objectives of the interviews are to

- collect information,

- verify and validate information obtained from other survey procedures, and

- provide the opportunity for all interested parties to provide what they believe is pertinent information.

These residents and family members will be asked specific questions to determine their satisfaction with the activity program.

- *How do you find out about the activities that are going on?*

- *Do you participate in activities?*

  -- *[If yes,] What kinds of activities do you participate in?*
  -- *[If resident participates,] Do you enjoy these activities?*
  -- *[If resident does not participate,] probe to find out why not.*

- *Is there some activity that you would like to do that is not available here?*

  -- *[If yes,] Which activity would you like to attend?*
  -- *Have you talked to anybody about this? What was the response?*

Interviews will continue with the resident council or an interviewable group of residents. Some of the questions that will be asked are:

- *Activity programs are supposed to meet your interests and needs. Do you feel the activities here do that? [If not, probe for specifics]*

- *Do you participate in the activities here? Do you enjoy them?*

- *Are there enough help and supplies available so that everyone who wants to can participate?*

- *Do you as a group have input into the selection of the activities that are offered? How does the facility respond to your suggestions?*

- *Is there anything about the activities program that you would like to talk about?*

- *Outside of the formal activity programs, are there opportunities for you to socialize with other residents?*

- *Are there places you can go when you want to be with other residents? [If answers are negative], Why do you think that occurs?*

Family interviews will be conducted by surveyors. Families will be asked to tell about the resident:

- *Did he/she enjoy any particular activities or hobbies?*
    - -- *Was he/she social or more solitary*
    - -- *Types of social and recreational activities*
    - -- *Religious/spiritual activities*
    - -- *Things that gave him/her pleasure*

- *Have her/his daily routines and activities changed in substantial ways since moving here? [If yes, please describe the differences.]*

E. Clinical Record Review

Clinical record review will assess the quality of care and quality of life that relate to the identified areas of concern for a resident. The purpose is to evaluate assessments, plans of care, and outcomes of care. The focus of the review is to determine if there has been a decline, improvement or maintenance in resident's functional abilities.

Surveyors will review clinical records of both current residents and discharged residents to evaluate if:

- Activities reflect individual resident history indicated by the comprehensive assessment;

- Care plans address activities that are appropriate for each resident based on the comprehensive assessment;

- Activities occur as planned; and

- Outcomes/responses to activities interventions are identified in the progress notes of each resident.

ASSESSMENT

KEY POINTS AND SUMMARY OF CHAPTER

Assessment is a coordinated process where all disciplines become involved in gathering information about the resident.

The Resident Assessment Instrument (RAI) which includes the Minimum Data Set (MDS) provides a framework for the assessment.

Section N Activity Pursuit Patterns is normally completed with input from the activity director.

A. Assessment Process

The purpose of a comprehensive assessment is to identify the resident's unique strengths, needs, preferences and potential for improvement. It allows the health professional to come to know the resident as an individual. Assessment answers the question: *Who is the resident?*

Comprehensive resident assessment provides the basis for care plan development to assure positive outcomes of care. Accurate and complete information sets up an environment for success. Delivery of quality health care is based on a process of gathering information about each resident in a systematic manner.

Interdisciplinary input to the assessment is gathered from various sources including the attending physician and other appropriate health professionals. Family members and the resident, if able, should be involved to identify resident preferences and family expectations.

COMPREHENSIVE ASSESSMENT SYSTEM:

Assessment
Gathering of information

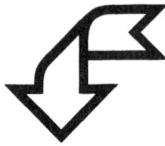

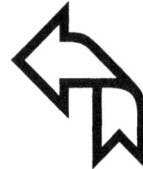

Decision-Making
*Identify problems and
underlying causes*

Evaluation
*Review resident's progress or
lack of progress toward goal*

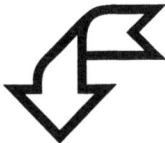

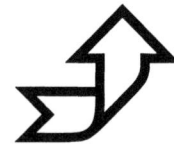

Goal Setting
*Establish attainable goals
for each problem*

Implementation
*Provide treatment
to the resident*

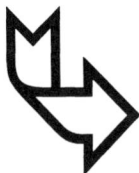

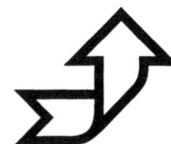

Interventions:
Action steps to be taken

Assessment information collected is used to develop the care plan. Once staff knows the resident, decisions are made on how best to provide care.

CARE PLAN PROCESS

Decision-making: Identification of resident problems, needs, and strengths and the underlying causal factors.

Goal setting: Establish realistic and attainable goals for each problem.

Interventions: Develop action steps for each health care discipline providing care to meet the established goals.

Each health care discipline is responsible for implementation of the action steps in the care plan. Based on the care plan, the activity professional documents the care provided in the clinical record. Forms such as behavior monitoring records, activity attendance records, one to one logs and other flow sheets contain documentation of interventions.

Periodically, a progress note is written to evaluate the care plan that describes:

- the success or lack of success in reaching the goals established in the care plan.

- resident response to the care plan.

Quarterly, each resident's care is reviewed at an interdisciplinary care conference. The resident's needs are re-evaluated. Problems, goals and approaches are updated. If care plan goals have not been reached or the resident's condition has changed, the approaches and interventions are revised. Use resident and family input to determine realistic expected outcomes for the care plan.

B. Federal Regulations

The resident assessment instrument (RAI) developed by CMS is completed by all nursing facilities participating in Medicare and Medicaid programs. The RAI includes a Minimum Data Set (MDS) and Resident Assessment Protocols (RAPs). The Resident Assessment Protocols (RAPs) contain utilization guidelines and triggers that provide a framework to translate the MDS data into an individualized care plan for the resident.

Completion of the Resident Assessment Instrument (RAI) is more than a paperwork exercise. By using common, universally-used definitions and coding categories, the MDS provides a systematic tool for gathering information to identify resident problems and conditions.

CFR Section 483.20 Resident Assessment

§483.20(b) Comprehensive Assessments.

(1)   Resident Assessment Instrument.   A facility must make a comprehensive assessment of a resident's needs, using the RAI specified by the State.   The assessment must include at least the following:

(i)   Identification and demographic information.
(ii)   Customary routine.
(iii)   Cognitive patterns.
(iv)   Communication.
(v)   Vision.
(vi)   Mood and behavior patterns.
(vii)   Psychological well-being.
(viii) Physical functioning and structural problems.
(ix)   Continence.
(x)   Disease diagnosis and health conditions.
(xi)   Dental and nutritional status.
(xii)   Skin conditions.
(xiii) Activity pursuit.
(xiv)   Medications.
(xv)   Special treatments and procedures.
(xvi)   Discharge potential.
(xvii) Documentation of summary information regarding the additional assessment performed through the resident assessment protocols.
(xviii) Documentation of participation in assessment.

(2)   When required, a facility must conduct a comprehensive assessment of a resident as follows:

(i)   Within 14 calendar days after admission, excluding readmissions in which there is no significant change in the resident's physical or mental condition. (For purposes of this section, "readmission" means a return to the facility following a temporary absence for hospitalization for therapeutic leave.)

(ii)   Within 14 days after the facility determines, or should have determined, that there has been a significant change in the resident's physical or mental condition. (For purpose of this section, a significant means a major decline or improvement in the resident's status that will not normally resolve itself without further intervention by staff or by implementing standard disease-related clinical interventions, that has

---

an impaction on more than one area of the resident's health status, and requires interdisciplinary review or revision of the care plan, or both.

(iii)   Not less than once every 12 months.

§483.20(c) Quarterly Review Assessment.

A facility must assess a resident using the quarterly review instrument specified by the State and approved by CMS not less frequently than once every 3 months.

§483.20(d) Use.

A facility must maintain all resident assessments completed within the previous 15 months in the resident's active record and use the results of the assessment to develop, review and revise the resident's comprehensive plan of care.

§483.20(g) Accuracy of Assessment.

The assessment must accurately reflect the resident status.

§483.20(h) Coordination.

A registered nurse must conduct or coordinate each assessment with the appropriate participation of health professionals.

§483.20(i) Certification.

(1)   A registered nurse must sign and certify that the assessment is completed.

(2)   Each individual who completes a portion of the assessment must sign and certify the accuracy of that portion of the assessment.

§483.20(j) Penalty for Falsification.

(1)   Under Medicare and Medicaid, an individual who willfully and knowingly—

(i)   Certifies a material and false statement in a resident assessment is subject to a civil money penalty of not more than $1,000 for each assessment; or

(ii)   Causes another individual to certify a material and false statement in a resident assessment is subject to a civil money penalty of not more than $5,000 for each assessment.

Additionally, the MDS is used to determine the amount of payment for Medicare Part A Prospective Payment System and for Medicaid payment in some states. Quality monitoring by CMS uses MDS data to calculate quality indicators used in the state survey process. Using MDS data, quality measures are posted on the internet website Nursing Home Compare (http://www.medicare.gov/NHCompare) so that consumers can access information about nursing homes.. Each professional contributing must complete the MDS accurately to assure the integrity of these CMS programs.

C.   Performing An Activity Needs Assessment

Activity pursuits are a need of all residents, not just those triggered by the MDS. By the very fact that the resident is in a nursing facility, their usual routines and leisure pursuits are no longer available to them. An activity needs assessment gathers information about how the resident wishes or is able to spend leisure time. The assessment should consider the residents normal every day routines and lifetime preferences.

CFR Section 483.20(b)(xiii) Guidelines

The facility is responsible for addressing all needs and strengths of residents regardless of whether the issue is included in the MDS or RAPs. The scope of the RAI does not limit the facility's responsibility to assess and address all care needed by the resident.

Activity pursuit (xiii) corresponds to MDS v2.0 Sections N and AC. Activity pursuit refers to the resident's ability and desire to take part in activities which maintain or improve, physical, mental, and psychosocial well-being. Activity pursuits refer to any activity outside of Activities of Daily Living (ADLs) which a person pursues in order to enhance a sense of well-being. Also includes activities which provide benefits in self-esteem, pleasure, comfort, health education, creativity, success, and financial or emotional independence. The assessment should consider the resident's normal everyday routines and lifetime preferences.

Promptly on admission, there must be an assessment of the resident by the activity professional to identify immediate needs, An admission care plan is developed to welcome the new resident, provide orientation and ease adjustment to the facility. The assessment process starts on admission and continues throughout the resident's stay.

The purpose of assessment is to identify appropriate activity pursuits that will enhance the quality of life for each resident. The activity assessment should consider the resident's normal everyday routine and lifetime preferences. Needs and strengths are identified and incorporated into the care plan.

Special considerations for activity assessment:

Cognition
Vision
Hearing
Communications abilities
Use of adaptive equipment
Pain
Foreign languages, cultural and religious backgrounds
Bedfast
New admission and welcoming activities

Evaluate information obtained first hand as well as input from the interdisciplinary care team. Direct observation and interview with the resident are the first steps to gathering information. A variety of information sources may be useful and could include licensed and non-licensed staff members including nurse aides on all shifts.

Other sources of information may include, but are not limited to:

*   attending physician,

*   family members,

*   direct care health professionals who have observed, evaluated, and/or treated the resident, and

*   the clinical record, including the admission record, physician's orders, documentation of services provided to the resident, reports of any diagnostic testing, consultation, or other services, medications administration record, copies of any transfer data provided by another health care facility and summaries of previous discharges.

Assessment information is documented in MDS Section N and a Supplemental Activity Assessment. The MDS collects basic information, but the MDS alone does not provide a comprehensive assessment. Supplemental assessments document the decision-making process by appropriate health care professionals of the scope of the resident's problems, needs or strengths that were triggered by the MDS. To be consistent, assessment must be made from objective and observable facts.

When assessment is performed correctly, it ensures that the plan of care is based on accurate and reliable information. A care plan based on the resident's unique needs improves the quality of life for the resident.

The activity assessment is a supplemental assessment of the resident. It includes the problems triggered by the MDS and information from the review of the Resident Assessment Protocols (RAPs) that were triggered by the MDS. This assessment utilizes information obtained not only in MDS Section N, but also from other sections of the MDS.

Elements of a Supplemental Activity Assessment		
Elements	**Assessment**	**MDS Item**
Physical	Diagnoses that limit resident function, such as cardiac dysrhythmia, hypertension, unstable/acute health conditions.	I J
Functional	Ability to walk, bedfast, wheelchair dependence, loss of hearing, visual impairments, need for hearing aid or glasses, amount of time awake.	C D G N
Mental Acuity/ Communications	Cognition, short or long term memory loss, length of attention span, ability to communicate needs, barriers to communication	B C
Social	Preferences regarding group activities, social interactions skills.	F
Psychological	Signs of distress, unsettled relationships, sadness over lost roles/status, inappropriate behavior, withdrawal.	E
Recreational values	Past likes and interest, expressed interest in more or different activities, little or no interest in diversional activities.	N
Spiritual	Religious affiliations & practices, meditation, reflection	N
Cultural	Ethnic customs, educational level, occupation, primary language other than English	Face Sheet
Customary Routines	Cycle of daily events, eating patterns, ADL patterns, involvement patterns	Face Sheet

D. Resident Assessment Instrument (RAI)

By using a systematic method, the health care professional can identify problems and needs unique to each resident. The Resident Assessment Instrument (RAI) which includes the Minimum Data Set (MDS) was designed as an interdisciplinary framework to minimize duplication of effort and strengthen team communication.

The RAI process includes the following:

- Minimum Data Set (MDS) as specified by each State,

- Triggers based on information completed in the MDS that identify resident assessment protocols that apply,

- Resident Assessment Protocols (RAPS) that contain description of problem, trigger logic and assessment guidelines,

- Utilization Guidelines developed by CMS on how to use the RAP for care plan development.

1. RAI Forms

The Resident Assessment Instrument includes the following forms:

- Tracking Form with Certification

- MDS Face Sheet

- Minimum Data Set (MDS)

- Resident Assessment Protocol (RAP) Summary

2. Time Frames

The RAI process is to be completed by the fourteenth (14) calendar day following admission. The day of admission is counted as Day 1. An MDS/RAI must to be completed for residents who stay longer than fourteen (14) days.

For residents who <u>do not</u> stay longer than 14 days, an MDS is <u>not</u> required. However, the facility must provide care appropriate for the resident's needs from admission through discharge regardless of length of stay. A modified MDS (MPAF) may be required for Medicare Part A residents who stay less than 14 days to determine payment for billing.

MDS SCHEDULE

Type of Assessment	Timing of Assessment
Admission Assessment (Initial)	Must be completed by the 14th day of the resident's stay
Annual Reassessment	Must be completed within 366 days of the most recent comprehensive assessment
Significant Change in Status Reassessment	Must be completed by the end of the 14th calendar day following determination that a significant change has occurred
Quarterly Assessment	Must be complete every 92 days

At least annually or if the resident experiences significant change, the resident assessment instrument must be redone. This includes MDS, triggers, RAPs and RAP summary. Each resident must have a comprehensive resident assessment no later than 366 days following the last comprehensive assessment. Some states may have additional requirements for the MDS completion.

Should a resident be transferred to an acute hospital and then return to the facility, determine if the resident has had a significant change in condition. A new comprehensive assessment is completed if the resident has experienced a significant change in status.

Do not conduct another assessment if the resident is readmitted and there has not been a significant change. However, for all readmissions, the immediate long or short-term activity needs must be re-evaluated even though there is no significant change.

3.   Quarterly MDS

Each resident's status is reviewed quarterly. Ideally, the quarterly MDS is completed and coordinated with an interdisciplinary team conference and the quarterly review of the resident care plan. A coordinated approach for completion of the quarterly MDS will provide continuity of assessment and efficient delivery of care.

The MDS quarterly review form is used to document a subset of *key items* required by federal regulations. Not all MDS items appear on the quarterly MDS. The form is numbered and scored in the same manner as the Minimum Data Set. Some States have an expanded quarterly assessment form or some States even require a full assessment on a quarterly basis.

Two items from Section N Activity Pursuits are included in the quarterly MDS :

- Time Awake (N1) and

- Average Time Involved in Activities (N2).

Comparison of quarterly assessment areas will assist with identifying any decline or improvement in a resident's functioning. If changes within the data elements indicate *significant change*, a complete RAI must be completed for the resident within fourteen (14) days.

If there have been changes in the resident's status that are not considered *significant change*, the appropriateness of the care plan is assessed. Goals are reviewed to determine if they are still realistic for the resident. If appropriate, changes in approaches and interventions are made to assist the resident to achieve the care plan goals.

4. Significant Change of Condition MDS

Each resident is examined and reassessed with the quarterly MDS. A comparison is made at this time to determine if there has been a significant change in condition of the resident that would require a new comprehensive MDS assessment under the regulations for significant change.

As part of the interdisciplinary team, activity professionals must be alert to indicators of significant change. A significant change of condition is defined as a major change in the resident's status that is not self-limiting, impacts on more than one area of the resident's health and requires interdisciplinary review or revision of the care plan.

Some indicators of significant change may include, but are not limited to, any of the following, or may be determined by a physician's decision, if uncertainty exists:

- Resident's decision making changes from 0 or 1 to 2 or 3 for B4 of the MDS. (*Consider whether activity programs are suitable for resident's cognitive level.*)

- Emergence of sad or anxious mood pattern as a problem that is not easily altered (E2 of the MDS). (*Perhaps resulting in refusal to attend activity programs*).

- Increase in the number of areas where behavioral symptoms are coded as (Eb4 = 1) not easily altered. (*i.e., an increase in the number of code (1) for E4b of the MDS*).

For example, Mr T no longer responds to verbal requests to alter his screaming behavior. It now occurs daily and has neither lessened on its own nor responded to treatment. He is also starting to resist his daily care, pushing staff away from him as they attempt to assist with his ADLs. The resident also has started to become disruptive in group activity programs. This is a significant change and reassessment is required since there has been a deterioration in the behavioral symptoms to the point where it is occurring daily and new approaches are needed to alter the behavior. Mr. T's behavioral symptoms could have many causes, and reassessment will provide an opportunity for staff to consider illness, medication reactions, environmental stress, and other possible sources of Mr. T's disruptive behavior.

The following are not considered significant changes:

• Discrete and easily reversible causes for which the facility staff can initiate corrective action.

• Short-term illness from which staff expects a full recovery.

• Well established, predictive cyclical patterns of clinical signs and symptoms with previously diagnosed conditions.

• If the resident continues to make steady progress under the current course of care, reassessment is required only when the condition has stabilized. However, if the facility is engaged in discharge planning, a reassessment is not required.

• In an end-stage disease status, a full reassessment is optional, depending on a clinical determination of whether the resident would benefit from it.

E.   MDS Rules for Completion

1.   Definitions

Uniform guidelines have been developed by CMS for completing the MDS. Because this system is used nationwide, it is important that health professionals use the same definitions and methods to collect data. The definitions are publishing in the Long Term Care Resident Assessment Instrument User's Manual that is published by CMS on the MDS 2.0 website (http://www.cms.hhs.gov/medicaid/mds20).

The MDS may be completed on paper form or entered directly into a computer. Certain rules for completing the MDS are as follows:

• Items with a letter in the answer box are completed with a check mark (Section N1, 3 and 4).

- Items that have a blank box are completed with a numeric response or a preassigned code (Section N 2 and 5).

- Complete all sections except when instructions specify to skip. In Section N Activity Pursuit Patterns after Item 1 Time Awake there is an instruction (If resident is comatose, skip to Section O).

- In cases where information is unavailable and despite continued probing, the information still remains unavailable, enter the code NA or a dash on computerized systems.

2. Assessment Reference Date

Section A Item 3 Assessment Reference Date (ARD) of the MDS is used to establish a common reference point for all data reported in the MDS. The assessment reference date (ARD) it is a specific end-point for a common observation period in the MDS assessment process.

Almost all MDS items refer to the resident's status over a designated time period referring back in time from the Assessment Reference Date (ARD) Item A3. Most frequently, the observation period is a 7 day period ending on the ARD. Some observation periods cover the 14 days ending on the ARD and some cover 30 days ending on the ARD.

In Section N Activity Pursuits there are five items. Each of the items have a seven (7) day look back period. This means that when Section N is completed, the information collected refers to a specific window of time, that is the seven days looking back from the Assessment Reference Date identified in Item A3.

The ARD is the seventh day of the observation period. Actual documentation of information on the MDS cannot start until the day after the Assessment Reference Date. The date for completion of the MDS and for certification of the MDS is after the ARD but on of before the actual required completion date of the MDS in Item R2b.

The Assessment Reference Date is not the date that the assessment documentation is completed. The ARD is scheduled by the RN Coordinator to assure that all items on the MDS reflect information from same period of time.

3. Section N Activity Pursuits

In most facilities, an activity professional will be responsible for completing Section N. Follow the MDS definitions carefully. Do not make up or change definitions.

Intent: To record the amount and types of interest and activities that the resident currently pursues, as well as activities the resident would like to pursue that are not currently available at the facility.

<u>Definition:</u>   Activity Pursuits. Refers to any activity other than ADLs that a resident pursues in order to enhance a sense of well-being. These include activities that provide increased self-esteem, pleasure, comfort, education, creativity, success, and financial or emotional independence.

The CMS <u>Long Term Care RAI User's Manual</u> provides the following guidelines for the completion of each item in Section N. Activity Pursuit Patterns.

Item N1.   Time Awake (7-day look back)

<u>Intent:</u>   To identify those periods of a typical day (over the last seven days) when resident was awake all or most of the time (i.e., no more than one hour nap during any such period).

For care planning purposes this information can be used in at least two ways:

- The resident who is awake most of the time could be encouraged to become more mentally, physically, and/or socially involved in activities (solitary or group).

- The resident who naps a lot may be bored or depressed and could possibly benefit from greater activity involvement.

<u>Process:</u>   Consult with direct care staff, the resident, and the resident's family.

<u>Coding:</u>   Check all periods when resident was awake all or most of the time.

a.   Morning - is from 7 a.m. (or when resident wakes up, if earlier or later than 7 a.m.) until noon.

b.   Afternoon - is from noon to 5 p.m.

c.   Evening - is from 5 p.m. to 10 p.m. (or bedtime if earlier).

d.   NONE OF ABOVE - If resident is comatose, code as "d", None of the above, and skip all other Section N items on the MDS and go to Section O on the MDS.

<u>Clarifications:</u> When coding this item, check each time period, as defined for that resident, during which he or she did not nap for more than one hour. Some examples of coding are as follows:

- A resident wakes up every morning at 7 a.m. He typically eats breakfast, has a shower, gets dressed and goes back to bed for a late morning nap from 10 a.m. until 11:30 a.m. Item N1a (Morning) should NOT be checked, since this resident typically naps for more than 1 hours during the morning.

- A resident typically wakes up at 6 a.m. She is busy with therapy and activities most of the day, and does not take naps. She goes to bed by 7 p.m. every evening. Items N1a (Morning), N1b (Afternoon) and N1c (Evening) should be checked, since this resident does not take naps.

- A resident who is bedfast and has end-stage Alzheimer's disease wakes up at 6 a.m. daily. She typically dozes off throughout the day, napping for more than 1 hour before noon, and again from 3:30 p.m. to 5:30 p.m. every afternoon. She is typically awake from 5:30 p.m. until 9 p.m. After that, she's asleep for the night. Items N1a (Morning) and N1b (Afternoon) should NOT be checked, since this resident naps for more than one hour during each of these periods. Item N1c (Evening) should be checked as time awake. Although this resident sleeps until 5:30 p.m., this is only a 30-minute nap time in the evening period.

Accurate coding relies on the use of appropriate information-gathering techniques. Coding Items N1a, b, and c based on only the assessor's personal knowledge of a resident's typical day may result in an inaccurate response to this item. Documentation review is important. However, we would generally not expect facility staff to maintain flowcharts for information such as sleep and awake times.

It is important to observe the resident across all shifts. In addition, the same individual staff member is generally not on duty and available to observe a resident across a 24-hour period. It's important to supplement observation with interviews of the resident, their family members, other staff across shifts, and in particular, the nursing assistants caring for the resident.

LEARNING EXERCISE FOR N1

Resident sleeps late until 9:00 a.m., stays awake until after lunch. Routinely this resident naps for 3 hours every afternoon and stays up in the evening to watch the 10 p.m. news on TV. Which time periods would be checked in Item N 1 Time Awake:

Morning	a___		Evening	c____
Afternoon	b___		NONE OF ABOVE	d____

Answer on Page 74

Item N2.   Average Time Involved in Activities (7-day look back)

Intent: To determine the proportion of available time that resident was actually involved in activity pursuits as an indication of overall activity involvement pattern. This time refers to free time when resident was awake and was not involved in receiving nursing care, treatments or engaged in ADL activities and could have been involved in activity pursuits and Therapeutic Recreation.

Clarification: Include the amount of free time a resident has while awake and is not involved in receiving nursing care, treatments, or engaged in ADL activities. Examples of activity pursuits and therapeutic recreation of his/her choice could include watering plants; reading; letter-writing; social contacts/visits or phone calls from family, staff, and volunteers; recreational pursuits in a group, one-on-one or on an individual basis; and involvement in therapeutic recreation. Keep in mind that the definition of *activity pursuits* refers to any activity other than ADLs that a resident pursues in order to enhance a sense of well-being. Efforts should be made to provide activities suited to the resident's preferences and capabilities.

Activity staff should work with cognitively impaired residents to identify what types of activities are suitable. Some impaired persons prefer to walk through the corridors rather than engaging in a seated activity. Based on the residents activity plan, certain activities, although not structured, may still be considered activities. The MDS Coordinator should work with the activities staff to determine which behaviors are considered appropriate activities for engaging the resident.

Many cognitively impaired persons continue to "pursue" their interests and also develop new interests. Activities must be tailored to their cognitive abilities. Record the amount of time the person spends in structured and non-structured activities.

Although dining is a social experience for some residents, and at times, meals may be planned around certain events or occasions, eating is not to be counted as an activity.

Process: Consult with direct care staff, activities staff members, the resident, and the resident's family. Ask about time involved in different activity pursuits.

Coding: In coding this item, exclude time spent in receiving treatments (e.g., medications, heat treatments, bandage changes, rehabilitation therapies, or ADLs). Include time spent in pursuing independent activities (e.g., watering plants, reading, letter-writing); social contacts (e.g., visits, phone calls) with family, other residents, staff, and volunteers; recreational pursuits in a group, one-on-one or an individual basis; and involvement in Therapeutic Recreation.

0.   Most-More Than 2/3 of Time
1.   Some-from 1/3 to 2/3 of Time
2.   Little-Less Than 1/3 of Time
3.   None

LEARNING EXERCISE FOR ITEM N 2

Resident is awake and dressed for 4 hours in the morning, takes a one-hour nap immediately after lunch and usually goes to sleep about 9:00 p.m. This resident has physical therapy daily for one hour, the family visits for 2 hours. Because the resident requires feeding assistance each meal take approximately one hour. The resident cannot attend the morning activity program because of the physical therapy treatments but does attend the 2 hour afternoon program.

How much time does the resident have available in the mornings for activities?   _____

How much time does the resident have available in the afternoon for activities?   _____

How must time does the resident have available in the evening for activities?   _____

   Total time available for activities   _____

How much time does the resident participate in activities each morning?   _____

How much time does the resident participate in activities each afternoon?   _____

How much time does the resident participate in activities each evening?   _____

   Total time participating in activities   _____

Code Item N 2 with the appropriate score: _____

0.   Most-more than 2/3 of time   1.   Some-from 1/3 to 2/3 of time
2.   Little-less than 1/3 of time   3.   None

Answer on page 74

Item 3.   **Preferred Activity Settings (7-day look back)**

Intent: To determine activity circumstances/settings that the resident prefers, including (though not limited to) circumstances in which resident is at ease.

Process: Ask the resident, family, direct care staff, and activities staff about the resident's preferences. Staff's knowledge of observed behavior can be helpful, but only provides part of the answer. Do not limit preference list to areas to which the resident now has access, but try to expand the range of possibilities for the resident. For example, ask the resident, *Do you like to go outdoors? Outside the facility (to a mall)? To events downstairs?* Ask staff members to identify settings that resident frequents or where he or she appears to be most at ease.

Coding: Check all responses that apply. If the resident does not wish to be in any of these settings, check NONE OF ABOVE.

     a.   Own Room
     b.   Day/Activity Room
     c.   Inside NH/Off Unit
     d.   Outside Facility
     e.   NONE OF ABOVE

LEARNING EXERCISE FOR ITEM N 3

Resident finds that the day room is too loud and noisy and has expressed a desire for in-room activities. This resident has a friend who is also a resident in another unit of the facility and does enjoy attending movies and music programs on the other unit in the company of the friend.

Check Item 3 with all that apply:

Own room   a._____   Day/activity room   b._____

Outside facility   d._____   Inside NH/off unit   c._____

NONE OF ABOVE   e._____

Answer on page 74

Item N4.   **General Activities Preferences (adapted to resident's current abilities) (7-day look back)**

Intent: Determine which activities, of those in the selected list, the resident would prefer to participate in (independently or with others). Choice is not limited by whether or not the activity is currently available to the resident, or whether the resident currently engages in the activity or not.

Definitions:

a.   **Cards/Other Games** – Activities involving games, such as trivia games.

b.   **Crafts/Arts**

c.   **Exercise/sports** -- Includes any type of physical activity (e.g. dancing, weight training, yoga, walking, sports, e.g., bowling, croquet, golf, or watching sports).

d.   **Music** -- Includes listening to music or being involved in making music (singing, playing piano, etc.)

e.   **Reading/writing** -- Reading can be independent or done in a group setting where a leader reads aloud to the group or the group listens to talking books. Writing can be solitary (e.g., letter-writing or poetry writing) or done as part of a group program (e.g., recording oral histories). Or a volunteer can record the thoughts of a blind, hemiplegic, or apraxic resident in a letter or journal.

f.   **Spiritual/religious activities** -- Includes participation in religious services as well as watching them on television or listening to them on the radio

g.   **Trips/Shopping**

h.   **Walking/Wheeling Outdoors**

i.   **Watching TV**

j.   **Gardening or plants** -- Includes tending one's own or other plants, participating in garden club activities, regularly watching a television program or video about gardening.

k.   **Talking or conversing** -- Includes talking and listening to social conversations and discussions with family, friends, other residents, or staff. May occur individually, in groups, or on the telephone; may occur informally or in structured situations.

l.   **Helping others** -- Includes helping other residents or staff, being a good listener, assisting with unit routines, etc.

m.   **NONE OF ABOVE**

Process: Consult with the resident, the resident's family, activities staff members, and nurse assistants. Explain to the resident that you are interested in hearing about what he or she likes to do or would be interested in trying. Remind the resident that a discussion of his or her likes and dislikes should not be limited by perception of current abilities or disabilities. Explain that many activity pursuits are adaptable to the resident's capabilities. For example, if a resident says that he used to love to read and misses it now that he is unable to see small print, explain about the availability of taped books or large print editions.

For residents with dementia or aphasia, ask family members about resident's former interests. A former love of music can be incorporated into the care plan (e.g., bedside audiotapes, sing-a-longs). Also observe the resident in current activities. If the resident appears content during an activity (e.g., smiling, clapping during a music program) check the item on the form.

Coding: Check each activity preferred. If none are preferred, check NONE OF ABOVE. Explore other possible sources of information, such as a responsible party that admitted the resident into the facility, or a surrogate decision maker who might know the resident's preferences. Is there any useful information in records that precede admission to the facility, such as hospital, community or home care records? If all resources are exhausted and you still do not have information, code the responses as information not available (-). If the resident appears content during an activity (e.g., smiling, clapping during a music program), check the item on the form.

LEARNING EXERCISE FOR ITEM N 4.

The resident has recently sustained a fractured hip and has a physician order for no weight bearing for 6 weeks. The resident has a television in the room, is an avid football fan, enjoys country music, often selects books from the library cart, and attends church services in a wheelchair.

Check Item N 4 with residents activity preferences.

Cards/other games	a.____	Trips/shopping	g.____
Crafts/arts	b.____	Walking/wheeling outdoors	h.____
Exercise/sports	c.____	Watching TV	i.____
Music	d.____	Gardening or plants	j.____
Reading/writing	e.____	Talking or conversing	k.____
Spiritual/religious Activities	f.____	Helping others	l.____
		NONE OF ABOVE	m.____

Answer on page 74

Item 5.   **Prefers Change in Daily Routines (7-day look back)**

Intent: To determine if the resident has an interest in pursuing activities not offered at the facility (or on the nursing unit) or not made available to the resident. This includes situations in which the activity is provided but the resident would like to have other choices in carrying out the activity (e.g., the resident would like to watch the news on TV rather than the game shows and soap operas preferred by the majority of residents; or the resident would like a Methodist service rather than the Baptist service provided for the majority of residents). Residents who resist attendance/involvement in activities offered at the facility are also included in this category in order to determine possible reasons for their lack of involvement.

Process: Review how the resident spends the day. Ask the resident if there are things he or she would enjoy doing (or used to enjoy doing) that are not currently available or, if available, are not right for him or her in their current format. If the resident is unable to answer, ask the same question of a close family member, friend, activity professional or nurse assistant. Would the resident prefer slight or major changes in daily routines, or is everything OK?

Coding: For each of the items, code for the resident's references in daily routines using the codes provided.

   0.   **No change** -- Resident is content with current activity routines

   1.   **Slight change** -- Resident is content overall but would prefer minor changes in routine (e.g., a new activity, modification of a current activity).

   2.   **Major change** -- Resident feels bored, restless, isolated, or discontent with daily activities or resident feels too involved in certain activities, and would prefer a significant change in routine.

LEARNING EXERCISES FOR ITEM N 5

Mrs. B is regularly involved in several small group activities. She also has expressed a preference for music. However, she has consistently refused to go to group sing-along when the activity staff offers to bring her. She says she doesn't like big groups and prefers to relax and listen to classical music in her room. She wishes she had a radio or tape player to do this.

Code Item N 5:   Code for resident preferences in daily routines
                   0. No change   1. Slight change   2. Major change

a.   Type of activities in which resident is currently involved   _____

b.   Extent of resident involvement in activities   _____

Answer on page 74

F. Certification of Accuracy of MDS

The RAI is best accomplished by an IDT that includes health care professionals who have clinical knowledge about the resident, including the activity professional. All health professionals contributing to the assessment must sign their full signature with professional title and date and indicate the section of the MDS that they completed in Item AA 9. Each person that completes information on the MDS is responsible for the accuracy of the items that were completed.

CFR Section 483.20(g) Accuracy of Assessment

Intent

To assure that each resident receives an accurate assessment by staff that are qualified to assess relevant care areas and knowledgeable about the resident's status, needs, strengths, and areas of decline.

Interpretive Guidelines

The accuracy of the assessment means that the appropriate, qualified health professional correctly documents the resident's medical, functional, and psychosocial problems and identifies resident strengths to maintain or improve medical status, functional abilities, and psychosocial status. The initial comprehensive assessment provides baseline data for ongoing assessment of resident progress.

*According to the Utilization Guidelines for each State's RAI, the physical, mental and psychosocial condition of the resident determines the appropriate level of involvement of physicians, nurses, rehabilitation therapists, **activities professionals,** medical social workers, dietitians, and other professionals, such as developmental disabilities specialists, in assessing the resident, and in correcting resident assessments. Involvement of other disciplines is dependent upon resident status and needs.*

Surveyors will look at clinical records to make sure that the appropriate certifications are in place, including the certification of individual assessors of the accuracy and completion of the portion(s) of the assessment tracking form or face sheet that they completed. Section AA9 (a) to (l) on the Basic Assessment Tracking Form contains signatures of persons completing portions of the MDS or tracking forms. Section AA9 contains the certification statement that staff members must sign and date attesting to the accuracy of the portions of the MDS completed by each member of the IDT. The signature and date of the person completing a section of the MDS must reflect that date that the documentation was completed. This date must be after the Assessment Reference Date (ARD) (A3) and on or before the MDS Completion Date (R2b) that is signed by the RN Coordinator as the date that the MDS was complete.

The certification statements is as follows:

I certify that the accompanying information accurately reflects resident assessment or tracking information for this resident and that I collected or coordinated collection of this information on the dates specified. To the best of my knowledge, this information was collected in accordance with applicable Medicare and Medicaid requirements. I understand that this information is used as a basis for ensuring that residents receive appropriate and quality care, and as a basis for payment from federal funds. I further understand that payment of such federal funds and continued participation in the government-funded health care programs is conditioned on the accuracy and truthfulness of this information, and that I may be personally subject to or may subject my organization to substantial criminal, civil, and/or administrative penalties for submitting false information. I also certify that I am authorized to submit this information by this facility on its behalf.

CFR Section 483.20(i) Certification

Interpretive Guidelines

Whether the MDS forms are manually completed, or computer generated following data entry, each individual assessor is responsible for certifying the accuracy of responses on the forms relative to the resident's condition . . . Manually completed forms are signed and dated by each individual assessor the day they complete their portion(s) of the MDS record. When MDS forms are completed directly on the facility's computer (e.g., no paper form has been manually completed), then each individual assessor signs and dates a computer generated hard copy, after they review it for accuracy of the portion(s) they completed. Backdating completion dates is not acceptable.

MDS information is used for multiple purposes that rely on accurate information. First of all, the MDS is used for the development of the resident care plan. Additionally, the MDS is used to determine the amount of payment for Medicare Part A Prospective Payment System and for Medicaid payment in some states. Quality monitoring by CMS uses MDS data to calculate quality indicators used in state survey process and quality measures that are posted on CMS's Internet Website Nursing Home Compare. Each professional contributing to the MDS must complete the MDS accurately to assure the integrity of these programs.

A pattern within a nursing home of clinical documentation or of MDS assessment or reporting practices that result in higher RUG scores, untriggering RAP(s), or unflagging QI(s), where the information does not accurately reflect the resident's status, may be indicative of payment fraud or avoidance of the quality monitoring process.

ANSWERS TO LEARNING EXERCISES

Item N (1)   a. Morning, c. Evening

Item N (2)

Hours available in morning	2
Hours available in afternoon	3
Hours available in evening	3
Total hours available	8
Morning activity time	0
Afternoon activity time	2
Evening activity time	2
Total activity time	4

1. Some -- 1/3 to 2/3 of time

Item N (3)   a. Own room, c. Inside NH/off Unit

Item N (4)   d. Music, e. Read/Write,
f. Spiritual Religious Activities, i. Watch TV

Item N (5)   a. 1 (Slight Change)
b. 1 (Slight Change)

Resident Assessment Protocols

....

KEY POINTS AND SUMMARY OF CHAPTER

Activity pursuits are a need for all residents, not just those triggered by the MDS.

Working the RAPs is a supplemental assessment process that links the MDS data to care planning.

Decision-making based on *working* the RAPs is essential for the development of a resident-centered care plan.

....

The Resident Assessment Protocols (RAPs) have been developed by CMS as a road map to guide the interdisciplinary team from assessment through care planning. *Working* the RAPs is an essential process to develop a resident specific care plan. The RAPs guide staff to identify underlying causes and unique risk factors that may be reversed or to prevent further deterioration.

There are eighteen (18) areas addressed by the resident assessment protocols (RAPs). One of the areas is Activities. However, activity professionals will find that many other RAPs include guidelines that impact the quality of the resident's life and activity pursuit. Some states have developed additional RAPs and CMS will continue to develop and revise RAPs to keep pace with changing clinical standards of care.

A. ₀Using the RAPS

The RAPs complete the Resident Assessment Instrument (RAI) by providing a problem-oriented format to transition to care planning. The RAPs are used to identify resident-specific problems, strengths and preferences and provide a decision-making guide for care plan development. The RAPs are not done with quarterly or Medicare MDS. RAPs are only completed with comprehensive assessments, such as, admission, annual and significant change of condition.

The RAPs contain four sections to assist the health professional in linking MDS data to care plan development:

- Problem,

- Triggers,

- Utilization Guidelines, and

- RAP Key.

Documentation in the clinical record must demonstrate that the health care professional used RAP guidelines. Supplemental assessments can be used to document the rationale or the thinking to proceed or not proceed with care planning. Thoughtful use of the guidelines in the RAPs will help staff identify ways to improve the outcome of care and ultimately the quality of life of residents in the nursing facility.

For example, a resident may be hard of hearing and the communications RAP is triggered. The RAP guidelines contain questions about risk factors and complications that would affect the resident's quality of life and activity participation. The interdisciplinary team assesses the causal factors to determine if they are reversible or how the hearing deficit will be managed. The activity professional uses the review of the RAP to develop an activity care plan that meets this resident's specific and unique needs related to the hearing deficit.

RAPs are not intended to regulate the method of providing care to the resident. The RAPs do not take the place of appropriate professional judgments. Rather, RAPs facilitate the understanding of potential problems, needs and strengths by directing health care professionals to consider specific guidelines when completing a supplemental assessment. The purpose of these guidelines is to assist the health care professional to identify the underlying causes and risk factors for each RAP triggered. By thoroughly assessing the underlying problem, a care plan can be developed that has the potential to reverse a problem or prevent further deterioration for the resident.

The complete text of CMS's Resident Assessment Protocol for Activity Pursuits can be found in the appendix of this book on page 169.

From the Long Term Care RAI User's Manual:

It is helpful to think of the RAI as a process. The MDS identifies actual or potential problems areas. The RAPs provide further assessment of the triggered areas; they help staff to look for causal or confounding factors (some of which may be reversible). Use the RAPs to analyze assessment findings and then chart your thinking. It is important that the RAP documentation include the causal or unique risk factors for decline or lack of improvement. A risk factor increases the change of having a negative outcome, or complication.

The RAPs will give the interdisciplinary team a sound basis for the development of the resident's care plan. After the comprehensive assessment process is completed, the interdisciplinary team will be able to decide if:

- *The resident has a troubling condition that warrants intervention, and if addressing this problem is a necessary condition for other functional problems to be successfully addressed;*

- *Improvement of the resident's functioning in one or more areas is possible;*

- *Improvement is not likely, but the present level of function should be preserved as long as possible, with rates of decline minimized over time;*

- *The resident is at risk for decline and efforts should emphasize slowing or minimizing decline, and avoiding functional complications (e.g., contractures, pain); or*

- *The central issues of care revolve around symptom relief and other palliative measures during the last months of life.*

B. Problem

Each RAP begins with a statement of the problem to be addressed. This is general information about how this RAP applies to a resident and the focus or objective of the care plan that is developed. For example, the problem statement for Activities RAP identifies four (4) types of activity pursuit needs or problems that are the objective and focus of the RAP guidelines. The RAP states that activity planning is a universal need for all residents. The specific focus of the RAP is to identify the resident for whom activity needs are not met or who have a condition the requires a review and reassessment of the activity plan.

> ### *From the Activities Resident Assessment Protocol*
>
> *For the nursing home (resident), activity planning is a universal need. For this (Activities) RAP, the focus is on cases where the system may have failed the resident, or where the resident has distressing conditions that warrant review of the activity care plan.*
>
> *The types of cases that will be triggered are:*
>
> *(1)   residents who have indicated a desire for additional activity choices;*
>
> *(2)   cognitively intact, distressed residents who may benefit from an enriched activity program;*
>
> *(3)   cognitively deficient, distressed residents whose activity levels should be evaluated; and*
>
> *(4)   highly involved residents whose health may be in jeopardy because of their failure to slow down.*

C.   Triggers

When marking certain items on the MDS form, resident problems, needs or strengths will be triggered. RAP triggers identify functional problems that may possibly be reversed or improved. Triggers are a method to flag conditions that need further assessment. With the help of the RAP guidelines, health care professionals make decisions whether or not the triggered condition should be addressed in the care plan.

When marking certain items on the MDS form problems/needs/strengths will be triggered. For example, marking Item N2 with (2) or (3) will indicate a trigger to consider revising the activity plan. Marking Item N2 with (0) will suggest a review of activity plan. The RAI system includes triggers as a method to identify conditions that need additional assessment.

Activity Triggers A identifies residents for whom a revised activity care plan may be required to identify those residents whose inactivity may be a major complication in their lives. Many will have ADL deficits, but few will be totally dependent. Impaired cognition will be widespread, but so will the ability to apply old skills and learn new ones. And sense may be impaired, but some type or two-way communication is almost always possible.

Activity Triggers B identifies residents now actively involved in activities for whom the activity care plan should be reviewed to assure that the plan remains appropriate for the resident. Of special interest are cardiac and other diseases that might suggest a need to slow down.

The MDS Training Manual gives the following example: Mrs. T is highly involved in activities of the facility. When structured activities are not scheduled, she keeps busy reading, crocheting and writing in a journal. Mrs. T awakens early in the morning and rarely takes a nap. MDS item Awake Mornings, N1a, is checked. MDS item Involved in Activities, N2, is coded 0 (most of time). Both of these MDS items are required to trigger the Activities RAP (Trigger B); these factors in combination suggest that the focus of the assessment should be on reviewing the current activities plan.

II. ACTIVITY TRIGGERS

Activity Triggers A (Revise)

<u>Consider revising activity plan if one or more of following present:</u>

    Involved in activities little or none of time [N2 = 2, 3]

    Prefers change in daily routine [N5a = 1, 2][N5b = 1, 2]

Activity Triggers B (Review)

<u>Review of activity plan suggested if both of following present:</u>

    Awake all or most of time in morning [N1a = checked]

    Involved in activities most of time [N2 = 0]

There are four different types of triggers that can influence the focus of a RAP review:

<u>Potential Problems:</u> These triggers suggest the presence of a problem for consideration and further assessment.

For example, Visual Function may be triggered and may be affecting the resident's ability to read a newspaper. Consultation for new eyeglasses and staff interventions to make sure that the resident's wearing of eyeglasses be made part of the care plan to assure increased participation and involvement in activity pursuits.

Broad Screening :

These are factors that assist staff to identify hard to diagnose problems.

Delirium and Dehydration are broadly defined triggers and will have a fair number of false positives. Experience has shown that these problems are often reversible but are difficult to recognize.

Prevention of Problems:

These are factors that identify residents who are at risk for developing particular problems.

For example, Activities Trigger B identifies residents who are currently fully participating in activities and should be reviewed to determine if they are at risk for over-stimulation.

Rehabilitation Potential:

Some triggers identify residents who can improve and identify resident strengths or minimize decline.

For example, a MDS item response indicates that the resident believes he or she is capable of increased independence in at least some ADLs (G8a). The assessment and care plan may focus on functional areas most important to the resident or on the areas with the highest potential for improvement. Activity exercise programs can be included on the care plan as interventions.

D.   Utilization Guidelines for Activities

When the Activity RAP is triggered, the RAP guidelines are reviewed to identify the nature of the problem and causal factors specific to the resident. The RAP is used as a tool to guide the assessment process so that information needed to fully understand the resident's condition is not overlooked. The information from the MDS and RAPs forms the basis for individualized care planning. The RAPs Summary form documents the decisions made during this evaluation process whether or not to proceed to care planning.

1.   RAP Key

The RAP Key provides an outline for evaluating data collected in the MDS. The RAP key is a quick reference but does not take the place of the main body of the RAP.

ACTIVITY RAP KEY

GUIDELINES

Issues to be considered as activity plan is developed:

- Time in Facility [AB1]
- Cognitive Status [B2, B4]
- Walking/Locomotion Pattern [G1c,d,e,f]
- Unstable Acute/Chronic Health Conditions [J5a,b]
- Number of Treatments Received [P1]
- Use of Psychoactive Medications [O4a,b,c,d]

Confounding problems to be considered:
- Performs Tasks Slowly and at Different Levels (Reduced Energy Reserves) [G8c,d]
- Cardiac Dysrhythmias [I1e]
- Hypertension [I1h]
- CVA [I1t]
- Respiratory diseases [I1hh, I1ii]
- Pain [J2]

Other issues to be considered:

- Customary Routines [AC]
- Mood [E1, E2] and Behavioral Symptoms [E4]
- Recent Loss of Close Family Member/Friend or Staff [F2f; from record]
- Whether or Not Daily Routine is Very Different from Prior Pattern in the Community [F3c]

Review of the RAP should include identifying why the RAP was triggered, that is what items on the MDS caused the RAP to trigger. This will steer the assessment process in the same direction as the focus and objectives of the RAP. This focused direction will be helpful in deciding if a care plan intervention is necessary, and what type of intervention is appropriate.

For example, the Activities RAP will trigger when item N2 Is scored 2 or 3, Involved in activities little or none of time.

The review of the RAP is intended to bring to light any associated factors about the resident's risks and potential complications. Knowing the trigger condition may clarify or possibly rule out certain approaches to the resident's problem.

---

2.   RAP Questions

The RAPs provide guideline questions to probe for additional clinically relevant information about an individual's health problems or functional status. The questions prompt the assessor to ask:

- What are the problems that require immediate attention?

- What risk factors are important?

- Are there issues that might cause you to proceed in a resident-specific manner for the RAP in question?

The Resident Assessment Protocol for Activities suggests some general questions that may be helpful in evaluating resident needs. Not all questions have to be addressed in RAP documentation, but they are guidelines to assist the activity professional to identify potential issues that need further assessment. The decision-making for the need to care plan is left up to the health professional.

From CMS Long Term Care RAI User's Manual

The RAP guidelines present comprehensive information for evaluation of factors that may cause, contribute to, or exacerbate the triggered condition. In addition to identifying causes or risk factors that contribute to the resident's problem, the guidelines assist the interdisciplinary team to:

- *Find associated causes and effects. Sometimes a problem condition (e.g., falls) is associated with just one specific cause (e.g., new drug that caused dizziness). More often, a problem (e.g., falls) stems from a combination of multiple factors (e.g., new drug, resident forgot walker, bed too high, etc.).*

- *Determine if multiple triggered conditions are related.*

- *Suggest a need to get more information about a resident's condition from the resident, resident's family, responsible party, attending physician, direct care staff, rehabilitative staff, laboratory and diagnostic tests, consulting psychiatrist, etc.*

- *Determine if a resident is a good candidate for rehabilitative interventions.*

- *Identify the need for a referral to an expert in an area of resident need.*

  - *Begin to formulate care plan goals and approaches.*

General Questions for all Residents

- *Is inactivity disproportionate to the resident's physical/cognitive abilities or limitations?*

- *Have decreased demands of nursing home life removed the need to make decisions, to set schedules, to meet challenges? Have these changes contributed to resident apathy?*

- *What is the nature of the naturally occurring physical and mental challenges the resident experience in every day life?*

- *In what activities is the resident involved?*

- *Is he/she normally an active participant in the life of the unit?*

- *Is the resident reserved, but actively aware of what is going on around him/her?*

- *Or is he/she unaware of surroundings and activities that take place?*

- *Are there proven ways to extend the resident's inquisitive/active engagement in activities?*

- *Might simple staff actions expedite resident involvement in activities?*

- *Can equipment be modified to permit greater resident access of the unit?*

- *Can the resident's location or position be changed to permit greater access to people, views, or programs?*

- *Can time and/or distance limitations for activities be made less demanding without destroying the challenge?*

- *Can staff modes of interacting with the resident be more accommodating, possibly less threatening, to resident deficits?*

Issues to be considered as activity plan is developed.

Is the resident suitably challenged?

- *Do available activities correspond to resident lifetime values, attitudes and expectations?*

- *Does resident consider "leisure activities" a waste of time -- he/she never really learned to play, or to do things just for enjoyment?*

- *Have the resident's wishes and prior activity patterns been considered by activity and nursing professionals?*

- *Have staff considered how activities requiring lower energy levels may be of interest to the resident -- e.g., reading a book, talking with family and friends, watching the world go by, knitting?*

- *Does the resident have cognitive/functional deficits that either reduce options or preclude involvement in all/most activities that would otherwise have been of interest to him/her?*

Confounding Problems to be considered

Health related factors that may affect participation in activities.

- *Is resident suffering from an acute health problem?*

- *Is resident hindered because of embarrassment/unease due to the presence of health-related equipment (tubes, oxygen tank, colostomy bag, wheelchair)?*

- *Has the resident recovered from an illness? Is the capacity for participation in activities greater?*

- *Has an illness left the resident with some disability (e.g., slurred speech, necessity for use of cane/walker/wheelchair, limited use of hands)?*

- *Does resident's treatment regimen allow little time or energy for participation in preferred activities?*

Other issues to be considered

Recent decline in status -- cognition, communication, function, mood or behavior.

- *Has staff or the resident been overprotective?*

- *Or have they misread the seriousness of resident cognitive/functional decline? In what ways?*

- *Has the resident retained skills, or the capacity to learn new skills, sufficient to permit greater activity involvement?*

- *Does staff know what the resident was like prior to the most recent decline?*

- *Is there any substantial reason to believe that the resident cannot tolerate or would be harmed by increased activity levels?*

- *Does resident retain any desire to learn or master a specific new activity? Is it realistic?*

- *Has there been a lack of participation in the majority of activities which he/she stated as preference areas, even though these types of activities are provided?*

Environmental factors.

- *Does the interplay of personal, social and physical aspects of the facility's environment hamper involvement in activities?*

- *Are current activity levels affected by the season of the year or the nature of the weather during the MDS assessment period?*

- *Can the resident choose to participate in or to create an activity? How is this influenced by facility rules?*

- *Does resident prefer to be with others, but the physical layout of the unit gets in the way?*

- *Do other features in the physical plant frustrate the resident's desire to be involved in the life of the facility?*

Changes in availability of family/friends support.

- *Has a staff person who has been instrumental in involving a resident in activities left the facility/been reassigned?*

- *Is a new member in a group activity viewed by a resident as taking over?*

- *Has another resident who was a leader on the unit died or left the unit?*

- *Is resident shy, unable to make new friends?*

- *Does resident's expression of dissatisfaction with fellow residents indicate he/she does not want to be a part of an activities group?*

Possible confounding problems to be considered for those now actively involved in activities.

- *Of special interest are cardiac or diseases that suggest a need to slow down.*

E.   Activity Program Related RAPs

Resident's strengths and needs in one area interrelate with strengths and needs in other areas. In addition to the information contained in Section N, other sections of the Minimum Data Set (MDS) will contain useful data for the development of the activity plan. Participation in the interdisciplinary team planning conference is an important step to integrate the activity plan with the comprehensive resident care plan. The activity professional will find that RAPs other than Activity Pursuit will require activity interventions and that activity interventions will be coordinated as part of care plans developed by other professional health disciplines.

Delirium	Delirium may be difficult to recognize and be mistaken for dementia. Delirium is never a part of normal aging.
Associated factors	• Psychosocial. Sad or anxious mood [E1, E2, E3], Isolation [F2e; from record], Recent loss [F2f], Depression [I1ee], Restraints [P4c,d, e,], Recent relocation [AB1;A4] • Sensory Impairment. Hearing [C1], Vision [D1]
Assessment	1. Identify possible underlying causes of delirium 2. Help screen for residents who have delirium for the purpose of treatment. • *Has the resident recently been admitted to a new environment (new room, unit, facility)?* • *Was there an orientation program that provided a calm, gentle approach with reminders and structure to help the new resident settle into the environment?* • *Has sensory deprivation led to confusion?* • *Has vision loss created sensory deprivation resulting in confusion?*
Care Plan	Any potential causes of delirium identified from this RAP review
Cognitive Loss/Dementia	Provide positive experiences for the resident (e.g., enjoyable activities) that do not involve overly demanding tasks and stress.
Confounding Problems	• Sensory impairment. Hearing problems [C1], Speech unclear [C5], Rarely/never understands [C6], Visual problems [D1]

Cognitive Loss/Dementia **Confounding Problems** **continued**	• Involvement factors. New admission [AB1], Withdrawal from activities [E1o], Participates in small group activities [F1f, N3b, record]
Assessment	1. To assist in identification of areas in which staff intervention might be beneficial 2. Provide appropriate care, enhance quality of life, sustain functional capacities, minimize declines, and preserve dignity.
Care Plan	• *Is resident willing/able to engage in meaningful communication?* • *Does staff use non-verbal communication techniques (e.g., touch, gesture) to encourage resident to respond?* • *Can resident participate more extensively in decisions about daily life?* • *Does resident retain any cognitive ability that permits some decision-making?* • *Is resident passive? Does resident resist care? Are activities broken into manageable subtasks?* • *Are residents with some cognitive skills and without major behavioral problems involved in the life of the facility and the world around them?* • *Are small group programs encouraged?* • *Are special environmental stimuli present (e.g., directional markers, special lighting)?* All measures to assist in developing a therapeutic environment for the resident with cognitive loss/dementia should be identified in the resident's care plan.
Visual **Issues and Problems**	Screen for presence of significant visual risk factors • Appropriate use of visual appliances [D3: from record, observation] • Environmental modifications [from record, observation]
Assessment	1. Review the resident's recent visual treatment history 2. Assist staff in determining if the visually impaired resident desires or has a need for increased functional use of the eyes.

Visual continued
Assessment
	3. Identify any acute visual problems and help accommodate any visual impairments.
	
	  • *Does resident report difficulty seeing TV/reading material of interest?*
	  • *Has the environment been adapted to resident's individual needs (e.g., large print signs marking room, color coded tape on dresser drawers, large numbers on telephone, reading lamp with 300 watt bulb)?*

Care Plan	Any visual risk factor, acute visual problem, or functional visual problem should be addressed in the resident's care plan with methods to ensure maximum visual function

Communication
 	
Confounding Problems
	Provide opportunities to communicate and accommodate the quality and quantity of communication.
	  • Decline in cognitive status [B6], increased mood problems [E3], decline in ADL status [G9]
	  • Hearing [C1], communication devices [C2, C3], decline in communication/ hearing [C7], vision [D1]

Assessment	1. The communication trigger suggests residents for whom a corrective communication treatment may be beneficial.
	2. Help staff develop both expressive and receptive means of communication for resident.
	
	  • *For chronic conditions that are unlikely to improve, consider communication treatments or interventions that might compensate for losses (e.g., for moderately impaired residents with Alzheimer's, the use of short, direct phrases and tactile approaches to communication can be effective)*
	  • *Are opportunities to communicate limited in ways (language) that could be remedied -- e.g., availability of partners?*

Communication continued **Care Plan**	The care plan should identify different means of communication such as verbal, written, sign language, gestures, communication boards, and/or observable resident behavior and affect that may assist the resident with receptive and expressive communication.
Psychosocial Well-Being **Confounding problems**	Identify resident who have problems with feelings about self and social relationships. • Increasing/persistent sad mood [E2, E3], increasing/daily disturbing behavior. • New admission [AB1, A4], change in room assignment [A2], daily routine is very different from prior pattern in the community [F3c] • Withdrawal from activities of interest [E1o]
Assessment	To assist in the identification of resident problems as they pertain to the resident's psychosocial well-being. • *Have key social relationships been altered/terminated (e.g., loss of family member, friend o staff)?* • *Do cognitive/communication deficits or a lack of interest in activities impede interactions with others?* • *Have changes in the resident's environment altered access to others or to routine activities -- for example, room assignment, use of physical restraints, assignment to new dining area?* • *Does resident indicate unease in social relationships?* • *Was life more satisfactory prior to entering nursing facility?* • *Is resident preoccupied with the past, unwilling to respond to the needs of the present?* • *Has the facility focused on a daily schedule that resembles the resident's prior lifestyle?*
Care Plan	The care plan should identify any areas that may be affecting the resident's psychosocial well-being with specific approaches to help the resident resolve these issues.

<u>**Mood State**</u> **Indicators of need**	Identify residents who have symptomatic signs of mood state problem. • Mood decline [E2] • Withdrawal from activities of interest [E1o] • Reduced social interaction [E1p]
Assessment	To assist staff in recognizing the causes and contributing factors involved with mood state problems. • *Has interest in activities declined, even though resident remains physically capable?* • *Does the resident show little/no initiative?* • *Does he/she remain uninvolved in activities (alone or with others)?*
Care Plan	The care plan should specifically identify the resident's mood(s) and how this mood affects the resident. Approaches should be listed to assist the resident in resolving issues that may be causing or exacerbating the mood problem.
<u>**Behavioral Problems**</u> **Potential causes**	Behavioral symptoms are often a source of danger and distress to the residents themselves and to other residents and staff. • Cognitive status problems. Delirium [B5], Alzheimer's Symptoms [I1q], or other dementia [I1u], • Effects of stroke [G5, G6, I1r, I1t] • Mood or relationship problems. Sad or anxious mood [E1], unsettled relationships [F2]. • Psychiatric diagnosis [I1dd, I1ee, I1ff, [I1gg] • Environmental conditions. Departure from resident's normal routines prior to entering facility [F3c], Staff responses, presence of stressful conditions of physically aggressive resident [from record; interviews with staff, resident] • Communications deficits. Difficulty making self understood [C4] or understanding others [C6] • Sensory impairments. Hearing problem [C1], Visual problem [D1]
Assessment	To assist staff in determining whether a resident's particular behavioral manifestation is an actual problem and to assist in the identification of potential causes or factors involved with these behaviors.

Behavioral Problems continued **Assessment**	• *Are staff sufficiently responsive? Do they recognize stressors for the resident and early warning signs of problem behavior?* • *Do staff follow the resident's familiar routines?* • *Do noise, crowding or dimly lit areas affect resident's behavior?* • *Are other residents physically aggressive?*
Care Plan	The care plan should identify specific resident behavioral symptoms and approaches to address these problems: a) qualitatively and quantitatively described resident behaviors; b) describe staff interventions when the resident exhibits the behaviors; and c) strategies to assist in preventing the resident's behavioral symptoms (such as meaningfully engaging activities, positive reinforcers, resident choices in care, etc)
Physical Restraints **Confounding problems**	Identify alternatives to restraint to enhance resident's quality of life • Sad/anxious mood [E1, Ea] • Resistance to treatment/meds and nourishments [E4e] • Unmet psychosocial needs [F1, F2, F3]
Assessment	Evaluate the potential use of restraints considering the resident's needs, problems, conditions, and risk factors which may justify the use of the restraint, if addressed, could reduce or eliminate the need for the restraint.
Care Plan	The care plan needs to address the reason for use of physical restraints as well as a restorative plan which may assist the resident to eventually discontinue use of the restraint. Many interventions (possibly involving activity programs) may be as effective or even more effective than restraints in managing a resident's needs, safety risks, and problems.

F. RAP Summary Form

The RAP Summary form is the final step in the comprehensive MDS. Each RAP triggered by the MDS data is identified and a decision to proceed or not proceed to care planning is recorded on the RAP Summary form. This form identifies problems triggered, decision to care plan and the location of the supplemental assessment information.

The instructions on the RAP Summary form state:

For each triggered RAP, use the RAP guidelines to identify areas needing further assessment. Document relevant assessment information regarding the resident's status. Documentation may appear anywhere in the clinical record (e.g., progress notes, consults, flow sheets, etc.) Indicate under the Location of RAP Assessment Documentation column where information related to RAP assessment can be found.

The RAP summary form is an index to those items triggered by the MDS. The RAP is reviewed for each problem triggered. From this review, a decision is made whether to proceed or not proceed to care planning. When a RAP is triggered, it simply means that additional assessment using the RAP Guidelines is required. It does not mean that a care plan must be developed for that particular condition.

All residents will have activity pursuit needs. However, not all residents will trigger the Activities RAP, even though activity pursuits are a universal need for residents in nursing facilities.

Identify only the RAP problems triggered by MDS information on the RAP Summary Form. Do not identify activity pursuits on the RAP summary form unless they are actually triggered, even though care planning will address all of the unique activity needs of the resident.

- Do not identify problems for the resident that are not triggered by the MDS. It is not an index to the all the problems on the care plan.

- Care plans may be written for other problems that are not identified through the MDS triggering process.

Finally, the location of the supplemental activity assessment information is identified. The location is usually in the activity assessment completed on admission. The facility may have other procedures for RAP narrative documentation such as specific narrative summary, computerized formats for RAP review, or elsewhere in the clinical record according to facility procedures. Be specific when identifying the location of supplemental assessment, including dates. Do not identify locations that do not contain assessment information. Do not duplicate or re-summarize information unnecessarily.

G. Documentation of the RAP Review

The RAP review process assists the activity professional to collect and analyze additional relevant information regarding the triggered condition. The guidelines also help to identify causal factors that affect the resident's condition and offer suggestions regarding how factors contributing to the resident's problems can be eliminated or minimized.

1. Content of RAP Documentation

The RAP Summary form can be thought of as a road map between the MDS and the care plan. The RAPs triggered by the MDS data identify suggested problems, needs or strengths of the resident. For each RAP triggered a decision is made whether or not to proceed to care planning. The location of the documentation of decision making is identified, such as, the supplemental activity needs assessment.

The decision-making process documents the causes and relationships between the residents problems and is a method used to understand the resident's needs. The supplemental assessment process includes documentation that the resident assessment protocols (RAPs) have been considered in the development of the care plan.

Documentation on the RAP Summary Form includes:

- The identification of the RAPs triggered by the data collection in the MDS.

- A determination of whether to proceed to care planning based on the information collected for each resident, and

- Location of summary information that documents review of the utilization guidelines and the decision-making process based on the Resident Assessment Protocols (RAPs).

The RAP summary documentation should describe:

- *Nature of the condition (may include presence or lack of objective data and subjective complaints).*

- *Complications and risk factors that affect the staff's decision to proceed to care planning.*

- *Factors that must be considered in developing individualized care plan interventions. Include appropriate documentation to justify the decision to care plan or not to care plan for the individual resident.*

- *Need for referrals or further evaluation by appropriate health professionals.*

Health care professionals use RAP guidelines to determine whether a new care plan is needed or whether changes will be made in the resident's existing care plan. In order to provide continuity of care for the resident and effective communication to all persons involved in the resident's care, it is important that information from the assessment that led the team to their care planning decision be clearly documented.

Documentation about the resident's condition should support clinical decision-making regarding whether or not to proceed with a care plan for a triggered condition and the type(s) of care plan interventions that are appropriate for a particular resident. It is not necessary to record all of the items referred to in the RAP Guidelines, such as, listing all factors that do and do not apply. Rather, documentation should focus on key issues, which may include:

- Why will you address or not address specific conditions in the care plan?

- How do the conditions affect the resident's daily functioning?

- Why did you decide the resident is at risk, or that improvement is possible, or that decline can be minimized?

- How could the resident benefit from consultation with an expert in a particular area (e.g., gynecologist, psychologist, surgeon, speech pathologist)?

Or, for triggered conditions that do not warrant care planning:

- Why did you determine that the triggered condition is not a problem for the resident?

2.   Locations of RAP Documentation

Documentation of the RAP review process may appear anywhere in the clinical record according to facility policy. Some appropriate locations are a narrative RAP summary, RAP Module, supplemental assessment forms and appropriately identified progress notes.

In most cases, the facility will have flexibility in documenting that the RAP has been *worked*. RAP documentation is a written account of the team's clinical thought processes about the resident assessment findings. Select the method or combination of methods that best fits with existing facility documentation practices.

Some computer programs will assist with this process by summarizing pertinent MDS items that apply to each RAP. This information can be useful as a worksheet for a RAP Narrative Summary. These worksheets can be used to demonstrate that the RAP guidelines have been reviewed. To complete the RAP documentation, simply add a narrative that describes the nature of the problem, risks and complications, care plan factors, referrals and rationale for care planning

RAP modules are often used and are mandated by some States. A RAP module lists questions contained in the RAP. A *yes, no* or *N/A* is completed to document that the utilization guidelines have been evaluated. RAP modules may be purchased from commercial forms vendors or may be produced by an MDS software program.

When using RAP modules, one must be aware that just answering the questions is not enough. Complete the RAP module with conclusions that described the problem identified, significant risk factors, factors to consider in care plan development, referrals and specify the rationale for proceeding or not proceeding to care planning.

Another option for documenting the RAP decision-making is to identify existing documentation in the chart. Depending on facility policy, this may be a less reliable method than other systematic options previously discussed. Problems arise in that there is no guarantee that all elements of the require RAP documentation summary have already been addressed in the record. Additionally, this can also be a time consuming task to identify these entries which, if not found, will require additional time spent in completing the documentation.

When identifying existing information already in the record, the location of information must be clearly identified with the date.

History and Physical 7/20/06

Nursing Admission Note 11/5/06

Activity Progress Note 2/16/06

Supplemental assessments such as the activity needs assessment will most likely contain the required documentation. Review supplemental assessment forms to assure that the content meets the utilization guidelines specified in the RAPs. When using supplemental assessment forms, clearly state the reason to proceed or not proceed to care planning.

Select a method of documenting the RAP process that fits with existing facility documentation procedures. The facility does not have to restrict themselves to one method. A combination of methods may be used on the same chart. Use methods that are routinely a part of your facility's clinical records. Examples of supplemental assessment forms are found in this book in Chapter 2, Selecting Forms.

H. Examples of RAP Documentation

The documentation of the RAP process can make a difference. Careful consideration of RAP Guidelines can assist health professionals to identify factors that can improve the quality of life of residents in a nursing facility. Time and again there is evidence that residents who would have fallen through the cracks were identified by the RAI process and poor outcomes of care avoided.

As the RAI has become an integral part of care delivery, many examples of successful interventions have been attributed to the RAI process. The following examples are two cases with similar MDS data but different underlying causes.

A resident triggered delirium and cognitive deficit. The review of the RAP determined that this is an established case of Alzheimer's dementia. A care plan was developed to promote self-sufficiency in a safe environment to enhance the quality of the resident's life, including a meaningful activity program specific to the resident's cognitive level.

Another resident also triggered delirium and cognitive deficit. However, the RAP review determined that the resident has diabetes that is out of control and has poor vision. By identifying the underlying causes, action steps were taken to stabilize those conditions. When the resident's diabetes came under control and he was properly oriented to the facility, the factors that triggered delirium and cognitive deficit disappeared. Activity programs were directed to orientation of the resident to daily activities and schedules. The room was arranged and self-help aids were made available. By identifying the resident's underlying problems, his quality of life was improved.

These example RAP assessments lead to two different care plans and two different outcomes. Consistent review of the RAP guidelines enables the health care professional to identify treatable underlying causes. Outcomes of care improve as skills in assessment improve. Problem identification and care plans driven by the RAP guidelines will lead to enhanced quality of life for each resident.

Care Plans

> **KEY POINTS AND SUMMARY OF CHAPTER**
>
> A comprehensive care plan is developed by the interdisciplinary team.
>
> An activity care plan is a universal need for all residents.
>
> The care plan identifies resident problems, unique characteristics, strengths and needs, sets time limited goals and specifies interventions that have been assigned to specific care givers.

A. Comprehensive Care Plans

A comprehensive care plan is essential for delivery of quality care and achievement of positive outcomes of care. The clinical record system hinges on this document. When all resident needs are identified and realistic goals set, the implementation of the plan will lead to the desired outcomes and quality of life for the resident. Unmet needs or unidentified problems can result in a decline in the resident condition and undesired outcomes of care.

Using the information gathered during the assessment process, a comprehensive plan of care is written with input from the interdisciplinary team. An appropriate care plan results from an analysis of consistent, reliable information, such as the data compiled by the MDS and other supplemental assessments. The benefit of a comprehensive care plan is that all caregivers are following the same interventions directed toward achieving common goals.

The interdisciplinary team develops a care plan that considers the resident's whole condition by:

- Identification of resident problems, unique characteristics, strength and needs,

- Establish goals,

- Set time limits in which to attain goals,

- Develop Interventions to reach goals, and

- Assign staff responsibility.

All residents have a need for activity planning, whether or not triggered by the MDS (Minimum Data Set). An activity care plan is a universal need for all residents. A care plan must be more than a paperwork exercise. It is a proven tool for delivering and improving resident care.

By the very fact that residents are in a nursing facility, they can no longer satisfy their need for diversional or recreational activities. They cannot go out to lunch with friends, shopping, to a theater or any other usual pursuits because of their physical requirements for hospitalization. It is the activity program's goals to identify residents' preferences and build on their strengths. Care plans are developed to supply meaningful diversions and stimulation within the facility environment.

B. Regulations for Comprehensive Care Plans

During the survey process, a sample of care plans will be reviewed. Surveyors will focus on the unique needs of each resident as identified in triggered RAPs, such as: cognitive deficit or intact, vision or hearing problems, communication or language barriers, and customary routines prior to admission. Section 483.20(k) of the federal regulations set the guidelines for evaluating compliance of comprehensive care plans.

CFR Section483.20(k) Comprehensive Care Plans

(k)   *Comprehensive care plans.*

(1)   *The facility must develop a comprehensive care plan for each resident that includes measurable objectives and timetables to meet a resident's medical, nursing, and mental and psychosocial needs that are identified in the comprehensive assessment.*

The plan of care must describe the following:

(i)   *The services that are to furnished to attain or maintain the resident's highest practicable physical, mental, and psychosocial well-being...*

(ii)   *Any services that would otherwise be required ... but are not provided due to the resident's exercise of rights ... including the right to refuse treatment.*

(2)   *A comprehensive care plan must be --*

(i)   *Developed within 7 days after the completion of the comprehensive assessment;*

(ii)   *Prepared by an interdisciplinary team, that includes the attending physician, a registered nurse with responsibility for the resident, and other appropriate staff in disciplines as determined by the resident's needs, and, to the extent practicable, the participation of the resident, the resident's family or the resident's legal representative; and*

(iii)   *Periodically reviewed and revised by a team of qualified persons after each assessment.*

Interpretive Guidelines: Section 483.20(k) Comprehensive Care Plans

An interdisciplinary team, in conjunction with the resident, resident's family, surrogate, or representative, as appropriate, should develop quantifiable objectives for the highest level of functioning the resident may be expected to attain, based on the comprehensive assessment. The interdisciplinary team should show evidence in the RAP summary or clinical record of the following:

-   *The resident's status in triggered RAP areas;*

-   *The facility's rationale for deciding whether to proceed with care planning and*

-   *That the facility considered the development of care planning interventions for all RAPs triggered by the MDS.*

The care plan must reflect intermediate steps for each outcome objective if identification of those steps will enhance the resident's ability to meet his/her objectives. Facility staff will use these objectives to monitor resident progress. Facilities

> *may, for some residents, need to prioritize care plan interventions. This should be noted in the clinical record or on the plan of care.*
>
> *The requirements reflect the facility's responsibility to provide necessary care and services to attain or maintain the highest practicable physical, mental and psychosocial well-being, in accordance with the comprehensive assessment and plan of care. However, in some cases, a resident may wish to refuse certain services or treatments that professional staff believe may be indicated to assist the resident in reaching his or her highest practicable level of well-being. Desires of the resident should be documented in the comprehensive assessment.*

The content of the care plan will be evaluated by surveyors to determine if the activity program is suitable for the individual resident.

For example:

• If a resident does not easily understand English, is it suitable for the resident to attend a News Talk program that is in English?

• If a resident has severely impaired vision, are radios or music part of their activity program?

• Is the activity program the appropriate level for enjoyment by a cognitively impaired resident?

• Are residents with short attention span placed close to the activity program's action in an attempt to stimulate them?

Surveyors also will determine if the care plan is carried out as planned. For example, activity attendance records will be checked to determine if the resident has attended suitable activities at the frequency identified in the care plan goal statement. Resident's will be observed to determine how their leisure time is being spent. Specifically, surveyors will look at residents who spend long hours without any apparently meaningful activity. Are they simply sitting in the hallways without being involved in any apparent type of meaningful activity?

Should a care plan not work or goals not met, the care plan needs to be adjusted and different approaches tried. For example, the activity care plan goals and interventions should be revised if the resident's attendance at group activity programs has decreased or the resident no longer participates actively or falls asleep during programs. To determine if a care plan is not working, review the care plan goals. If the goals are not being met, the approaches in the care plan should be reviewed and new approaches developed.

A reassessment of the resident must be documented that evaluates any underlying causal factors that may contribute to the lack of success of the care plan. Such reassessments may be completed quarterly during the regular review of MDS information or at anytime in between when it is identified that the goals of the care plan are not being met or there is a significant change in condition.

Survey Procedures and Probes:
Section 483.20(k) Comprehensive Care Plans

Does the care plan address the needs, strengths and preferences identified in the comprehensive resident assessment?

Is the care plan oriented toward preventing avoidable declines in functioning or functional levels?

How does the care plan attempt to manage risk factors?

Does the care plan build on resident strengths?

Does the care plan reflect standards of current professional practice?

Do treatment objectives have measurable outcomes?

Corroborate information regarding the resident's goals and wishes for treatment in the plan of care by interviewing residents, especially those identified as refusing treatment.

Determine whether the facility has provided adequate information to the resident so that the resident was able to make informed choices regarding treatment.

If the resident has refused treatment, does the care plan reflect the facility's efforts to find alternative means to address the problem?

Is the care plan evaluated and revised as the resident's status changes?

Residents have the right to refuse to participate in activity programs. However, the resident should be assessed to determine the reasons that the resident does not wish to participate. Alternate activities, such as in room music and books, should be provided as well as assessing family or other significant support that involves the resident with meaningful leisure time.

If the resident's refusal results in a significant change, the interdisciplinary team should reassess the resident and institute care planning changes. For example, if a resident refuses to leave his or her room and exhibits symptoms of depression, the care plan could be revised with interventions, such as, psychiatric consult, and drug and non-drug interventions to manage depression.

C. Procedures for Care Planning

A plan is developed which outlines the care to be given, the objectives to be accomplished and the professional discipline responsible for each element of care. The care plan should be initiated on admission for any immediate needs. A comprehensive care plan is completed seven (7) days following the completion of the resident assessment instrument (RAI).

A care plan is at the heart of daily care delivery and improving the quality of the resident's life in the facility. Using the information gathered by assessment, a care plan is a blueprint for meeting the needs of the resident.

Periodically, the resident care plan is reviewed, evaluated and updated by the health professionals involved in the care of the resident. At a minimum the plan is reviewed quarterly by the interdisciplinary team and coordinated with each minimum data set (MDS) assessment. The care plan is revised more often if there is a change in the resident's condition or the goals of the care plan are not achieved.

PROCEDURE FOR WRITING CARE PLANS

1. On admission a resident care plan is started with all known immediate problems and needs for the resident. For the activities program input to the care, welcoming and orientation needs should be addressed.

2. A comprehensive care plan is developed for each resident that includes measurable objectives and timetables to meet a resident's medical, nursing and mental and psychosocial needs that are identified through the comprehensive assessment process.

3. The resident's problems and needs are identified from those triggered by the Minimum Data Set, review of the physician's orders for services to be provided or withheld and input from supplemental assessments of other appropriate staff in disciplines determined by the resident's needs. All resident need activity input to the care plan, even though the Activities RAP did not trigger. Activity plans are a universal need for all residents.

4. The Resident Care Plan includes input from all professionals involved in the

---

care of the resident. When practical, the resident, the resident's family or the resident's legal representative are provided an opportunity to contribute to the care plan.

5.   Short Term Goals (Objectives) are identified for each problem in measurable, observable terms. Goals provide a mechanism for evaluating resident progress.

6.   A realistic time limit in which to accomplish each goal is established. If a problem is of an ongoing nature, indicate "q 3 months" as the time limit.

7.   Care to be given (interventions) specify methods to be implemented to accomplish the objective for each problem.

8.   The professional discipline responsible for each intervention is identified.

9.   The professional entering the problem signs their initials and verifies the initials with the full signature.

10.   As the resident's condition or capacity changes, the resident care plan is updated. The date indicates when a new problem was identified and care planned.

11.   After each quarterly MDS assessment, the plan is reviewed, evaluated and updated by the all professional personnel involved in the care of the resident.

12.   The date of each quarterly review is indicated on the resident care plan.

13.   When a problem is resolved, a yellow highlighter pen is used to mark through the problem. The word "Resolved" and the date are recorded.

14.   Skip at least two lines between each problem to allow for updating and additional input.

15.   The care plan is written in ink or generated by computer. The care plan is a part of the resident's clinical record.

D.   Problem Identification

Following the completion of the Resident Assessment Instrument (MDS) and the supplemental assessments, all information about the resident is reviewed. The MDS will trigger or identify certain problems that need to be addressed in the care plan. From the composite of all information known about each resident, problems and needs are identified. However, the MDS is a minimum data set and will not trigger all of the resident's problems and needs. These additional problems and needs will be identified by the inter-disciplinary team through the supplemental assessment process. Remember that activities is a universal need for all residents in a nursing facility.

Writing the resident's needs on the care plan is an important first step. Style issues are secondary. Needs can be listed as problem statements, RAP titles, nursing diagnoses, medical diagnoses or any other format that staff understands. When a need is identified, staff should be encouraged to write it down, regardless of the words used. Federal regulations do not contain a required format or mandated terminology.

Problems/needs statements have two components:

- First a description of the problem/need stated in functional or behavioral terms.

- Second is the underlying cause to identify the physical and/or mental limitations and/or strengths.

Examples of problem statements are:

Diversional activity deficit due to confusion and short attention span and inappropriate group behavior (hitting others)

Needs in-room activities due to non-weight bearing status following hip surgery and severe pain.

From Long Term Care RAI User's Manual

When the interdisciplinary team has identified problems, conditions, limitations, maintenance levels or improvement possibilities, etc., they should be stated, to the extent possible, in functional or behavioral terms (e.g., how is the condition a problem for the resident; how does the condition limit or jeopardize the resident's ability to complete the tasks of daily life or affect the resident's well-being in some way.

EXAMPLES

- *Mr. Smith cannot find his room independently*

- *Mrs. Jones slaps at the faces of direct care staff while they are giving personal care.*

- *Mr. Brown is unable to walk more than 15 feet because of shortness of breath.*

EXAMPLES OF PROBLEM STATEMENTS

Description of Problems, Strengths or Needs	Underlying Cause (due to) (related to)
Complaints of boredom, loneliness	removal from normal interpersonal and social contact
Constant demands and irritability	refusal to accept limitations or participate in rehabilitation efforts
Decreased participation in activity programs	visual impairment hearing deficit foreign language
Decreased strength/mobility	arthritis, pain, lack of motivation
Diversional activity deficit	decreased stamina, loss of mobility, confusion and short attention, inappropriate group behavior, refuses to participate
Lack of social interaction	withdrawal from social contact, lack of motivation, refuses to participate in activities
Limited interaction with others	expressed preference for room activities only
Needs in-room, bed appropriate activities	non weight bearing status
Non-responsive to environment	cerebral vascular accident
Short attention span and restlessness	cognitive deficit, noise intolerance
Uncooperative/ disruptive behavior	Mental confusion, inability to communicate needs
Withdrawal from social and interpersonal interactions	recent loss of loved one, relocation to nursing facility

E.   Setting Goals

Based on the resident assessment, long term and short term goals are developed. A long term goal identifies the expected outcome for the resident's stay. Short term goals identify the expected results of care provided. Goals are dynamic and may be changed frequently as the resident progresses or regresses

1.   Long Term Goals

Long-term goals address the expected outcome of the hospitalization and are general in nature. Residents in nursing facilities have three general types of long-term goals:

- Rehabilitative goals that expect a resident to return to a previous level of functioning or a higher level of functioning.

- Maintenance goals that expect a resident to remain at the same level of functioning and not deteriorate.

- Supportive goals to keep the resident comfortable for those who are terminal or have a progressive disease process.

2.   Short term Goals

Each individual problem on the care plan should have a goal to address the immediate expectations to be achieved. Once a short-term goal is achieved, a new more ambitious goal can be developed if appropriate. The key to successful care planning is setting realistic, resident-oriented goals that are attainable for the resident

Realistic goals answer the questions:

- Can the resident achieve the goal with his/her functional limitations?

- How will resident's strengths help achieve the goal?

Resident oriented goals answer the questions:

- Does the resident want to achieve the goal?

- Is this outcome desired by the resident and family?

It is helpful when writing resident-centered measurable goals to ask: *How do we know it is a problem?* The answer will lead to a measurable goal: *Because she will not attend group activities.*

3.   **Goal Statements**

Objectives or goals are written in measurable terms. A measurable goal is a phrase or statement by which the resident's progress can be evaluated in objective terms by any knowledgeable health care professional. A measurable goal specifies the amount of time and level of involvement of the resident in activities of his or her choice.

Subjective (Not Measurable): Resident will be less depressed

Objective (Measurable):   Resident will select three (3) group activities to participate in each week (if the depression resulted in withdrawal from social contact.)

Goals should include, whenever possible, resident strengths. Strengths may include: adequate vision, motivation for getting well, participation of family or friends.

Goals are an expression in objective and realistic measurements of the expected outcome of the planned interventions. The goal statements include:

• What activity or behavior is desired,

• A standard of objective measurement, and

• Time frame within which to accomplish the desired outcome of care.

The terminology for stating goals has three parts. First, identify what outcome is expected or desired. Next describe what measurement will determine if the resident has achieved the goals. And finally, how long will it take to reach the goals.

The format of the goal statement would be:

Identify outcome: The resident will participate in at least __#__ activities per week (specify which activities).

Indicate the
Desired Outcome: Responds to questions
State name when asked
Make eye contact during activity
Track ball with eyes
Hit ball when directed toward self
Sing/mouth words to song
Keep time to music with rhythm instrument

State time limit for goal: Date to be accomplished

---

1.   **Terminology for interventions**

The interventions or approaches are statements of actions and steps that will be done to help the resident in achieving the stated goal. Identify specific services to be offered.

A format for the approaches should be:

• Arrange attendance at (specify which activities)

• 1:1 visits (specify activity, i.e., conversation, tactile stimulation, sensory stimulation)

• Involve family/volunteer (how, i.e., take resident out of facility once a week, read correspondence to resident)

For example, an approach can be written as:

Activity Director will invite resident to attend Thursday afternoon music program. Resident will be asked to participate in selection of music.

Responsibility for the interventions can be documented in several ways:

• include in the approach/intervention a statement that

Activity Director will
by social worker
by certified nursing assistant

• include in the care plan form a column to identify responsible discipline

---

From CMS Long Term Care RAI User's Manual

Specific, individualized steps or approaches that staff will take to assist the resident to achieve the goals(s) will be identified. These approaches serve as instructions for resident care and provide for continuity of care by all staff. Short and concise instructions, which can be understood by all staff, should be written.

The goals and their accompanying approaches are to be communicated to all direct care staff who were not directly involved in the development of the care plan. Communication about care plan changes should be ongoing among interdisciplinary team members.

EXAMPLES OF INTERVENTIONS

Actions to be taken	Specific services
Attend arts and crafts weekly	remind resident to finish project
Escort to morning exercise	praise resident for effort
Active participation	in resident council
Attend happy hour	offer snacks and nourishments
Volunteer visit weekly	take outside to garden assist in tending potted plants
Provide careful supervision during craft classes	be alert that resident may place items in mouth
Family visit every evening	to assist with feeding dinner
Include in reality orientation group	address resident by first name
Provide communication board	engage in conversation
Counsel resident regarding angry outbursts	encourage discussion of feelings
Counsel resident regarding inappropriate language	praise resident for efforts
Arrange attendance at dieter's support group	encourage verbal participation
No morning activity participation	allow resident to sleep in
Provide small watering can	for tending indoor plants in room
Place in front row for movies	be sure that hearing aid is working and resident is wearing glasses

G. Care Plan Conference

The care plan is based upon the information collected in the Minimum Data Set as well as information gathered by the interdisciplinary care team. The plan is started at the time of admission for the resident's immediate needs. The comprehensive care plan is developed by the interdisciplinary team within seven (7) days of completion of the resident assessment instrument.

At a minimum the interdisciplinary team should include the licensed nurse responsible for the resident, the certified nursing assistant assigned to the resident, the **activity director**, social worker and dietitian or dietary manager. If the resident is receiving restorative therapy, the therapists should attend.

Although it is not required that an attending physician attend the interdisciplinary team conference, the physician should review that care plan to assure that it is appropriate for the resident. This may be indicated by signing approval on the care plan or by writing an order that the care plan has been reviewed and approved.

To assure that the activity plan is not in conflict with the physician's treatment plan, it is good practice to request physician orders for:

a.   use of alcoholic beverage,

b.   deviations from therapeutic diet,

c.   permission to leave facility for outing, and/or

d.   ability to participate in physical exercises programs.

When setting goals, resident and family cooperation and understanding is needed so all may work toward a common end. Participation by the resident or resident's family/legal representative is essential for the success of care planning. The care plan should be resident-oriented and include opportunities for the resident to exercise choice and self-determination, whenever possible. Do not underestimate the potential for success and positive outcomes that result from resident and family involvement in care planning.

Interpretive Guidelines: Section 483.20(k)(2) Interdisciplinary Team

As used in this requirement, interdisciplinary means that professional disciplines, as appropriate, will work together to provide the greatest benefit to the resident. It does not mean that every goal must have an interdisciplinary approach. The mechanics of how the interdisciplinary team meets its responsibilities in developing an interdisciplinary care plan (e.g., a face to face meeting, teleconference, written

---

communication) is at the discretion of the facility.

The physician must participate as part of the interdisciplinary team, and may arrange with the facility for alternative methods, other than attendance at care planning conferences, of providing his or her input, such as one-to-one discussions and conference calls. . .

The facility has a responsibility to assist residents to participant, e.g., helping residents, and families, legal surrogates or representatives understand the assessment and care planning process; when feasible, holding care planning meetings at the time of day when a resident is functioning best; planning enough time for information exchange and decision making; encouraging a resident to attend (e.g. family member, friend) if desired by a resident.

The resident has the right to refuse specific treatments and to select among treatment options before the care plan is instituted. The facility should encourage residents, surrogates, and representatives to participate in care planning, including encouraging attendance at care planning conferences if they so desire.

While federal regulations affirm the resident's right to participate in care planning and to refuse treatment, the regulations do not create the right for a resident, legal surrogate or representative to demand that the facility use specific medical intervention or treatment that the facility deems inappropriate. Statutory requirements hold the facility ultimately accountable for the resident's care and safety, including clinical decisions.

Survey Procedure and Probes: Section 483.20(k)(2) Interdisciplinary Team

- *Was interdisciplinary expertise utilized to develop a plan to improve the resident's functional abilities?*

- *Is there evidence of physician involvement in development of the care plan (e.g., presence at care planning meetings, conversations with team members concerning the care plan, conference calls)?*

- *In what ways do staff involve residents and families, surrogates, and/or representatives in care planning?*

- *Do staff make an effort to schedule care plan meetings at the best time of the day for residents and their families?*

- *Do facility staff attempt to make the process understandable to the resident/ and family?*

> • *Ask residents whether they have brought questions or concerns about their care to the attention of facility's staff? If so, what happened as a result?*
>
> • *Is the care plan evaluated and revised as the resident's status changes?*
>
> • *Do care plans address activities that are appropriate for each resident based on the comprehensive assessment?*

H. Interdisciplinary Care Plan

Coordinated team planning is essential for meeting all of the resident needs and achieving good outcomes. Although the activity professional has the lead responsibility in the development of the activity plan based on the Activities RAP, input and responsibility will be appropriate in several other RAP areas.

The care plan complex consists of the problem statement, the goals and the approaches. In some facilities, each discipline writes their own problem complex. However, more than one discipline may need to provide input regarding the same problem. An interdisciplinary problem complex includes input from all appropriate disciplines to the problem statement, the goals and the approaches. More than one discipline may be identified as responsible for implementing the plan.

The Long Term Care RAI User's Manual states that the team may find during their discussions that several problem conditions have a related cause but appear as one problem for the resident. Or they may find that they stand alone and are unique. Goals and approaches for each problem condition may be overlapping, and consequently the interdisciplinary team may decide to address the problems conditions in combination on the care plan.

Interdisciplinary input can be accomplished in two ways:

• Each discipline has a clearly identified problem complex written in each care plan

• Each discipline contributes causal factors to the problem statements, goals unique to their discipline, and approaches they plan to implement or recommend. Each discipline would initial the input to the various problem complexes to which they contributed.

For example, the activity professional will provide input and include activity plan approaches for problems identified by several of the RAPs.

Delirium   Delirium is a symptom of a variety of acute, treatable illnesses. Even with successful treatment of cause(s) and associated symptoms, it may take several weeks before cognitive abilities return to pre-delirium status.

Problem and Goal Statement	Interventions (by Activities)

Delirium
as evidenced by
    disorderly thinking
related to
    recent surgery
    pain medication
 	
Goal:
    will be oriented to time, place and person by two weeks
    pain level will be reduced to mild pain daily by Day 5
	Ensure access to clock and calendar in room
	
	One to one visits twice a day to reorient to time, place and person
	
	Bring to music programs 3 times a week
	
	Ask family to bring radio or CD player for in room soft music.

Cognitive Loss/Dementia   One of the three main goals of this RAP is to develop care plans that provide positive experiences for the resident, such as enjoyable activities, that do not involve overly demanding tasks and stress.

Problem and Goal Statement	Interventions (by Activities)

Cognitive Decline
as evidenced by
    short term memory loss
related to
    Alzheimer's disease
 	
Goal:
    will participate in two activities daily
    will make choices between two options
	Assist with selection of menu items giving resident choices between two items
	
	Activities of interest are
	    painting class
	    sing along
	    excursions out of facility once a week
	    pet visit by volunteers
	
	Family visits twice a week in evenings

<u>**Visual Function**</u>

Residents with visual problems may have difficulty identifying small objects and enjoying certain activities programs. Such difficulties can cause a resident to become cautious and ultimately refuse to participate in activity programs.

The consequences of vision loss are wide-ranging and can seriously affect physical safety, self-image, and participation in social, personal, self-care and rehabilitation activities.

Problem and Goal Statement	Interventions (by Activities)

<u>Impaired vision</u>
as evidenced by
    unable to read but can see large images
    can see adequately for safe ambulation
related to
    macular degeneration, progressive
 	
<u>Goal:</u>
    will not injure self or others when ambulating
    will verbalize fears re sight
	Adapt environment to maximize visual functions
	    large print signs
	    large numbered phone
	    night light
	
	Volunteer to read romance novels to resident three times a week.
	
	Attend activities twice a day for current events, movies, music.
	
	Escort to activity locations

<u>**Communications**</u>

Good communication enables residents to express emotion, listen to others, and share information. It also eases adjustment to a strange environment and lessens social isolation and depression.

As language use recedes with dementia, both the staff and the resident must expand their nonverbal communication skills -- one of the most basic and automatic of human abilities. Touch, facial expression, eye contact, tone of voice and posture all are powerful means of communicating with the demented resident, and recognizing and using all practical means is the key to effective communication.

Details of resident strengths and weakness in understanding, hearing, and expression are the direct or indirect focus of any treatment program.

For chronic conditions that are unlikely to improve, consider communication treatments or interventions that might compensate for losses (e.g., for moderately impaired residents with Alzheimer's, the use of short, direct phrases and tactile approaches to communication can be effective)

Problem and Goal Statement	Interventions (by Activities)
Communication impaired as evidence by difficulty in understanding conversations related to hard of hearing speaks limited English, foreign language primary (Spanish) Goal: will understand simple sentences in English	Speak in short simple phrases. Address resident from the left side which is the good ear. Have family or interpreter available for medical care discussions Attend activities twice a day music painting pets

Psychosocial Well-Being

Well-being refers to feelings about self and social relationship. Positive attributes include initiative and involvement in life; negative attributes include distressing relationships and concern about loss of status.

Well-being problems or needs to maintain psychosocial strengths are suggested if there is withdrawal from activities of interest or if the daily routine is very different from prior pattern in the community.

Well-being strengths are suggested if the resident establishes own goals or there is strong identification with past.

Resident can withdraw or become distressed because they feel life lacks meaning. Activity programs are the main opportunity in nursing facilities for residents to socialize and provide meaning to life.

Problem and Goal Statement	Interventions (by Activities)
<u>Adjustment to facility</u> as evidenced by 　　expresses uneasiness about staying in facility and expresses wish to go home related to recent admission <u>Goal:</u> 　　will participate in one daily activity of choice for first month 　　will verbalize positively to roommate within next 7 days	Refer to social worker for possible discharge planning Make sure activity calendar is available and invite to activity program every day If does not attend a program, follow up with one to one visit to determine if special interests can be accommodated. Provide TV schedule for sports events

Mood State　　Consider a problem if withdrawal from activities and/or reduced social interaction.

The passive resident with distressed mood may be overlooked. Such a resident may be erroneously assumed to have no mood state problem

Problem and Goal Statement	Interventions (by Activities)
<u>Mood decline</u> as evidenced by 　　insomnia related to 　　depression <u>Goal:</u> 　　sleep 6-8 hours each night	Provide PM snack of warm milk after resident has prepared for bed Participation in evening activity program at least 3 times a week

Behavior　　Care plan development for residents who exhibit the behavioral symptoms of wandering, being verbally abusive, being physically aggressive and/or exhibiting socially inappropriate behavioral symptoms.

Some resident may not be capable of meaningful communication. However, many of the seemingly incomprehensible behaviors (e.g., screaming, aggressive behavior) in which these individuals engage may constitute their only form of communication. By observing the behavior and the pattern of its occurrence, one can frequently come to some understanding of the needs of individuals. For example, residents who are restrained for their own safety may become noisy due to bladder or bowel urgency.

Use non-verbal communication techniques (e.g., touch, gesture) to encourage resident to respond.

Problem and Goal Statement	Interventions (by Activities)

Behavioral symptoms
as manifested by
    wandering and attempting to leave the facility
related to
    Alzheimer's dementia
 	
Goal:
    will participate in 2 activity programs
    will not injure self or leave the facility without supervision
	Make sure resident attends afternoon activity programs since this is the time she is most restless.
	
	Include in activities that are physically active such as exercise group
	
	One to one volunteer will take resident out on patio and walks in garden
	
	Include resident in excursions outside of the facility

Nutritional status

Residents with loss of appetite may be helped by programs involving food preparation and that include refreshments.

Residents who are fearful, who pace or wander, withdraw from activities, cannot communicate, or refuse to communicate, often refuse to eat or will eat only a limited variety and amount of foods.

Problem and Goal Statement	Interventions (by Activities)

Nutritional status altered
as manifested by
    recent 5% weight loss
related to
    decreased appetite
 	
Goal:
    will maintain weight or gain back weight loss
	Involve in activities relating to food such as cooking class on Thurs
	
	Offer snack during programs such as popcorn, juices and cookies
	
	Encourage family to bring in foods that the resident likes. Store appropriately at nursing station.

<u>**Restraints**</u>   Many interventions may be as effective or even more effective than restraints in managing a resident's needs, safety risks and problems.

Problem and Goal Statement	Interventions (by Activities)

<u>Needs Lap Cushion</u>
to prevent resident from slipping out of
    wheelchair
related to
    weakness due to old CVA
 	
<u>Goal:</u>
 	
    will be able to sit comfortably and
    safely in wheelchair during afternoons
    no falls or injury from wheelchair
	Resident will be up every afternoon and attend activities he prefers such as
	    art class
	    music programs
	    pets
	    sports on television
	
	Reposition resident every 2 hours
	
	CNA to toilet resident prior to bringing to afternoon activity program

Progress Notes

> ### KEY POINTS AND SUMMARY OF CHAPTER
>
> Progress notes evaluate the resident's response and the results of the implementation of the care plan.
>
> Progress notes should be written at least quarterly and more frequently if the resident has a significant change in condition.

Progress notes evaluate the outcome of the care plan. They are the final step of the documentation process. Good clinical progress notes communicate relevant and essential information in a concise manner. The resident's condition is described and response to interventions is observed in measurable terms. The activity professional must have the ability to identify clinically and/or legally significant events that require narrative documentation.

The purpose of progress notes is to:

- evaluate the resident's response to the plan of care and treatment.

- document the progress, maintenance or regress in respect to the goals identified in the care plan.

When writing progress notes, the problems and needs of the resident that are identified in the care plan must be reviewed. The progress notes describe the resident's response to the interventions in the care plan. Any discrepancy between what is actually happening and what was planned needs to be clarified at this time. The assessment, the care plan and the progress notes must agree in content.

A. Steps for Writing Progress Notes

Before writing a progress note follow these steps:

- Observe the resident's response to activity interventions.

- Discuss the resident with other professional staff to identify any changes in condition.

- Review physician orders for new or discontinued orders that may influence the resident's activity level.

- Review attendance records and flow sheets to identify subtle changes in resident behavior.

- Review previous progress notes to evaluate if the resident has changed or goals have not been met.

- Update the care plan if resident's activity level has changed.

B. Content of Progress Notes

Activity progress notes are written at least quarterly to evaluate the resident's progress, regress or maintenance of the goals specified in the care plan. A progress note must be accurate, objective and complete.

Descriptions should be specific to the resident's condition. Observe for objective findings. Describe what is seen. If the resident makes subjective statements, record them as *Resident states that . . .*

Avoid terms that are nonspecific. For example, *usually, frequently, at times or occasionally* are not measurable. Measurable documentation will state the number of times, how many times, what time something occurs.

The content of a progress note evaluates the goals identified in the care, response to interventions and treatments and any new or short-term problems. Progress notes must be concise. Do not repeat a description of the care plan. Do not repeat information contained elsewhere in the health record unless there is more explanation needed.

Progress notes document the results of the care plan:

- How did the resident respond or adjust to the placement in the facility?

- How does the resident interact with staff and other residents?

- What is the resident doing now that he or she did not do in the past?

- Did an intervention not produce the anticipated result?

- Record the degree of success or lack of success in attaining a specific goal.

- How has the resident changed since the care plan was written? Are there any new or short-term goals?

- What actions have been taken to resolve problems and how has the resident responded?

- Is the resident satisfied with the activity program?

OUTLINE FOR PROGRESS NOTES

Activity Participation	Usual attendance pattern
	Special events attended
	Level of participation
One to One needs	Motivation/socialization
In room activities	Family involvement
Resident Response	Satisfaction with programs offered
Outcomes	Progress, regress or maintenance of care plan goals
MDS assessment	Significant change in
	Mentation
	Communication/hearing
	Vision Changes
	Mood/behavioral symptoms
	ADL function
	New diagnosis
	End of Life
	Nutrition/weight loss

C.   Flow Sheets

Flow sheets are used to document resident information to be compared over a period of time. Flow sheets may be used to document activity program interventions and level of participation. Such flow sheets with information pertinent to the activity program may include:

Attendance records

One to one visit logs

Flow sheets enable the activity professional to document and review data in a quick and efficient manner. Also when evaluating the resident's condition, data can be easily found and compared. Use flow sheets to track resident participation in activity programs over time. Attendance logs will indicate frequency of participation or identify trends such as refusing to attend certain activities.

Review all flow sheets to gather information prior to the quarterly interdisciplinary team conference and to assist in writing the quarterly activity progress note.

D.   Timing of Progress Notes

Quarterly narrative notes are written by the activity program staff to evaluate in descriptive terms the progress or lack of progress toward the goals set in the care plan. Identify new problems as they occur and evaluate the resident's response to care and treatment.

Establish a schedule for writing quarterly progress notes. Spread the work over a period time so each resident can be evaluated individually. It is most efficient to coordinate the writing of quarterly progress notes with the interdisciplinary team conference.

Be alerted to the quarterly update of the minimum data set. Any significant change or deterioration in the resident's activity of daily living skills may change a resident's level of participation in the activity program.

Meaningful and informative progress notes shall also be written as often as the resident's condition warrants.

- If the resident's condition changes

- On readmission following a temporary discharge to evaluate any change in the resident's activity needs

- At any more frequent intervals as specified by state regulations

If a resident is readmitted to the facility from the acute hospital, the activity director must assess the resident's activity status at that time. Often level of participation will change, if only temporarily following hospitalization. The resident may have lost strength in the hospital due to the acute illness. There may be a new diagnosis, medications or treatments or a change in functional level or mental acuity that will require an alteration of the activity plan.

Resident and Family Council

9

The Resident and Family Council provides an opportunity for choice and self-determination. By discussing and offering suggestions, the resident or family member can influence the quality of their life in the facility and resident and family satisfaction with the care provided.

Key steps in attaining resident and family satisfaction are:

- participation in care planning,

- attendance at resident and family councils,

- ability to make choices, and

- mechanism to voice grievances.

A. Federal Regulations

Section 483.15 (c) of the federal regulations provide for resident/family groups to discuss care and life in the facility and make recommendations.

CFR Section 483.15(c) Resident and Family Groups

(c)   Participation in resident and family groups.

    (1)   A resident has the right to organize and participate in resident groups in the facility;

    (2)   A resident's family has the right to meet in the facility with the families of other residents in the facility;

    (3)   The facility must provide a resident or family group, if one exists, with private space;

    (4)   Staff or visitors may attend meetings at the group's invitation;

    (5)   The facility must provide a designated staff person responsible for providing assistance and responding to written requests that result from group meetings;

    (6)   When a resident or family group exists, the facility must listen to the views and act upon the grievances and recommendations of residents and families concerning proposed policy and operational decisions affecting resident care and life in the facility.

Interpretive Guidelines: Section 483.15(c) Resident/Family Council

This requirement does not require that residents organize a residents or family group. However, whenever residents or their families wish to organize, facilities must allow them to do so without interference. The facility must provide the group with space, privacy for meetings, and staff support. Normally, the designated staff person responsible for assistance and liaison between the group and the facility's administration and any other staff members attend the meeting only if requested.

A residents or family group is defined as a group that meets regularly to:

- Discuss and offer suggestions about facility policies and procedures affecting residents' care, treatment, and quality of life;
- Support each other;
- Plan resident and family activities;
- Participate in educational activities; or
- For any other purpose.

The facility is obligated to listen to resident and family group recommendations and grievances. Acting upon these issues does not mean that the facility must accede to all group recommendations, but the facility must seriously consider the group's recommendations and must attempt to accommodate those recommendations, to the extent practicable, in developing and changing facility policies affecting resident care and life in the facility. The facility should communicate its decisions to the resident and/or family group.

B. Resident Group Interview

One of the tasks of the survey process is the resident group interview. If a resident and/or family council exists, the surveyors will meet with these groups for the interview task.

Survey Procedures: On Site Preparatory Activity Task2 B2

The (surveyor) team coordinator or designee should contact the resident council president after the Entrance Conference to introduce him/herself and to announce the survey. Provide the president with a copy of the group interview questions. Request the assistance of the president for arranging the group interview and to solicit any comments or concerns. Ask the council president for permission to review council minutes for the past 3 months.

If there is not an active resident council, or if the council does not have officers, ask for a list of residents who attend group meetings, if any, and select a resident representative to assist in arranging the group interview. If the ombudsman has indicated interest in attending the group interview, ask the president if that is acceptable to the group; if it is, notify the ombudsman of the time/place of the meeting.

The questions asked by the surveyors are a resident or family satisfaction survey. These same questions can be used by the facility for review with resident or family councils on a regular basis as part of the facility's Quality Assessment and Assurance program. By interviewing residents and families in this method, problems can be identified early and resolved quickly. Such interviews improve public relations and provide a feeling of control or empowerment for those involved in the interviews.

The survey process requires that group interviews are conducted and specifies the following set of questions on CMS Form 806B Quality of Life Assessment Group Interview.

QUALITY OF LIFE ASSESSMENT GROUP INTERVIEW

RULES:

Tell me about the rules in this facility.

For instance, rules about what time residents go to bed at night and get up in the morning?

Are there any other facility rules you would like to discuss?

Do you as a group have input into the rules of this facility?

Does the facility listen to your suggestions

PRIVACY:

Can you meet privately with your visitors?

Can you make a telephone call without other people overhearing your conversation?

Does the facility make an effort to assure that privacy rights are respected for all residents?

ACTIVITIES:

Activities programs are supposed to meet your interests and needs. Do you feel the activities here do that (If no, probe for specifics)

Do you participate in the activities here?

Do you enjoy them?

Are there enough help and supplies available so that everyone who wants to can participate?

Do you as a group have input into the selection of the activities that are offered?

How does the facility respond to your suggestions?

Is there anything about the activities program that you would like to talk about?

Outside of the formal activity programs, are there opportunities for you to socialize with other residents?

Are there places you can go when you want to be with other residents? (If answers are negative) Why do you think that occurs?

PERSONAL PROPERTY:

Can residents have their own belongings here if they choose to do so?

What about their own furniture?

How are your personal belongings treated here?

Does the facility make efforts to prevent loss, theft, or destruction of personal property?

Have any of your belongings ever been missing?

(If anyone answers yes) Did you talk to a staff member about this? What was their response?

RIGHTS:

> *How do residents here find out about their rights -- such a voting, making a living will, getting what you need here?*
> *Are you invited to meetings in which staff plans your nursing care, medical treatment and activities?*
> *Do you know that you can see a copy of the facility's latest survey inspection results?*
> *Where is that report kept here?*
> *Do you know how to contact an advocacy agency such as the ombudsman office?*
> *Do you know you can look at your medical record?*
> *Have any of you asked to see your record? What was the facility's response?*
> *Has anyone from the facility staff talked to you about these things?*
> *Tell me about the mail delivery system here. Is mail delivery prompt? Does your mail arrive unopened daily?*

DIGNITY:

> *How do staff members treat the residents here, not just yourselves, but others who can't speak for themselves?*
> *Do you feel the staff here treat residents with respect and dignity?*
> *Do they try to accommodate resident's wishes where possible?*
> *(If answers are negative) Please describe instances in which the facility did not treat you or another resident with dignity. Did you talk to anyone on the staff about this? How did they respond?*

ABUSE AND NEGLECT:

> *Are you aware of any instances in which a resident was abused or neglected?*
> *Are you aware of any instances in which a resident had property taken from them by a staff member without permission? (If yes) Tell me about it. How did you find out about it?*
> *Are there enough staff here to take care of everyone? (If no) Tell me more about that.*
> *We are willing to discuss any incidents that you know of in private if you would prefer. If so, just stop me or one of the other surveyors anytime, and we'll listen to you.*

COSTS:

> *Are residents here informed by the facility about which items and services are paid by Medicare or Medicaid and which ones you must pay for?*
> *If there was any change in these items that you must pay for, were you informed?*

Are you aware of any changes in the care any resident has received after they went from paying for their care to Medicaid paying?
(If answers suggest the possibility of Medicaid discrimination, probe for specific instances of differences in care)

BUILDING:

I'd like to ask a few questions about the building, including both your bedroom and other rooms you use such as the dining room and activities room.
Is the air temperature comfortable for you?
Is there good air circulation or does it get stuffy in these rooms?
What do you think about the noise level here? Is it generally quiet or noisy? How about at night?
Do you have the right amount of lighting in your room to read or do whatever you want to do?
How is the lighting in the dining rooms and activity rooms?
Do you ever see insects or rodents here" (If yes) Tell me about it.

FOOD:

The next questions are about the food here.
Is the flavor and appearance of your food satisfactory?
Outside of the dietary restrictions some of you may have, do you receive food here that you like to eat?
If you have ever refused to eat a particular food, did the facility provide you with something else to eat? (If no, probe for specifics)
If the temperature of your hot and cold foods appropriate?
Are the meats tender enough?
About what time do you receive your breakfast, lunch and dinner?
Are the meals generally on time or late?
What are you offered for a bedtime snack?
If you ever had a concern about your food, did you tell the staff? What was their response?

COUNCIL:

Does the facility help you with arrangements for council meetings?
Do they make sure you have space to meet?
Can you have meetings without any staff present if you wish?
How does the council communicate its concerns to the facility?
How does the administrator respond to the council's concerns?
If the facility cannot accommodate a council request, do they give you a reasonable explanation?

GRIEVANCES:
Have any of you or the group as a whole ever voiced grievance to the facility?
How did staff react to this?
Did they resolve the problem?
Do you feel free to make complaints to staff? If not, why not (probe for specific examples)?

It is recommended that these questions are periodically asked of the resident council to evaluate and identify problems. This could be done by taking one set of questions for discussion at each monthly meeting.

C.   Minutes

Meetings are most productive when effectively organized. The activity professional can assist the resident or family council in setting up an agenda prior to the meeting.

Minutes of resident and family councils are necessary for meetings to be meaningful. Writing the minutes may be part of the assistance provided by staff. Often this duty is part of the activity professional's job description.

Minutes should include:

Date

Time of meeting

Names of persons attending

Unresolved issues and status

Resolved issues and action taken

New concerns

Follow up to ongoing issues

Signature of person taking the minutes

SAMPLE NURSING FACILITY

MINUTES OF RESIDENT COUNCIL

Date_____

The meeting was called to order by the Chairman, (Name) at (time) am/pm.

The following residents attended the meeting:

The following staff members or guests were invited to attend the meeting:

The minutes of the previous meeting were reviewed and approved.

The following unresolved issues were discussed and reports were given of action taken in response to the issues raised by the Resident Council.

The following issues were resolved by (specify the action taken to resolve each issue).

The following new issues were discussed and recommendations were made.

The meeting was adjourned at (time) am/pm.

Respectfully submitted,

Secretary

SAMPLE NURSING FACILITY

RESIDENT COUNCIL ACTION SUMMARY

FOR THE MONTH OF _____

PROBLEMS	ACTION	RESOLUTION

Submitted by_____, Activity Director

Reported to_____, Administrator

D. Action Summary

In addition to narrative minutes a summary sheet to follow up issues raised at the resident council is helpful to document that facility has seriously considered any recommendations and has made attempts to accommodate these recommendations. This action summary should track the issues, actions taken and follow up.

EXAMPLE OF RESIDENT COUNCIL ACTION SUMMARY

PROBLEMS	ACTION	RESOLUTION
Suggest birthday parties be held on weekends or evenings so families could attend	Activity Director will survey families to determine most convenient time	Report to January meeting
Request warm drinks for nourishments on winter afternoons in November through March	Activity Director will contact the Dietary supervisor to discuss. Possibility to purchase microwave discussed with Administrator	Warm drink is now available on Unit I. Microwave purchased in November Unit II will have microwave by February

Quality Assessment and Assurance

10

```
••••••••••••••••••••••••••••••••••••••••••••••••
```

KEY POINTS AND SUMMARY OF CHAPTER

Quality Assessment and Assurance (QAA) is an ongoing program and not just a once a year crash effort to prepare for survey.

A QAA program matches expected outcome of care to actual practice to find opportunities for improvement.

Quality indicators are measurements of outcomes of care.

Audit checklists are used to determine compliance and identify problem areas the need to be improved.

```
••••••••••••••••••••••••••••••••••••••••••••••••
```

Quality Assessment and Assurance (QAA) is a continuous program that monitors the ability of a nursing facility to achieve positive outcomes of care. A QAA program matches expected outcomes of care to actual practice. When expectations are not met, staff is alerted that potential problems exist.

The result of an effective quality assessment and assurance program is identification and resolution of problems before they become too large or too difficult to fix. Early identification of trends provides opportunities to improve resident care.

A. Federal Regulations

CMS has made a commitment not only to survey for compliance with regulations but also to improve the quality of care in nursing homes. MDS data is used to calculate quality indicators that are used in the survey process. These indicators measure and identify potential areas of concern. Quality measures are also posted on the CMS website Nursing Home Compare. Consumers can access the site for information about nursing homes. The federal regulations require that nursing homes have a process to review and improve quality of care. Specifically, a QAA Committee must be functioning in the facility.

CFR Section 483.75(o) Quality Assessment and Assurance Committee

(1)   A facility must maintain a quality assessment and assurance committee consisting of

    (i)   The director of nursing service;

    (ii)   A physician designated by the facility;

    (iii)   At least 3 other members of the facility staff.

(2)   The quality assessment and assurance committee

    (i)   Meets at least quarterly to identify issues with respect to which quality assessment and assurance activities are necessary; and

    (ii)   Develops and implements appropriate plans of action to correct identified quality deficiencies.

(3)   A State or the Secretary may not require disclosure of the records of such committee except in so far as such disclosure is related to the compliance of such committee with the requirements of this section.

During the survey process, the quality assessment and assurance protocol will be reviewed by the surveyor to determine that:

•   A Quality Assessment and Assurance Committee exists and meets at least quarterly.

•   The committee has a method, on a routine basis, to identify, respond to, and evaluate its response to issues which require quality assessment and assurance activity.

Because QAA reports and minutes are confidential, surveyors may not review the documentation. To determine that there is an effective QAA program, surveyors may ask QAA committee members and/or direct care staff questions about the QAA committee.

Direct care staff should know how to access the QAA process and committee. Access may be by participation on the committee or by submitting reports. Staff will attend inservice training in response to problems identified by QAA.

B. Implementation

To implement a QAA program, each facility must develop a system to measure actual performance and identify areas for improvement. Action is taken to correct any deficiencies found. And finally, evaluate and follow up to assure that problems have been solved and quality improved.

Dr. W. Edward Deming was a pioneer in the development of quality assurance methods. His system outlined the following steps:

Plan:
Study existing processes to decide if change will lead to improvement. Set a specific objective and measurable outcome to be attained. Identify who, what, where, when and how the study will be done.

Do:
Measure actual practice against expected practice outcomes. Identify problems and procedures that need change.

Study:
Check and evaluate the results and draw conclusions.

Act:
Implement policy and procedure changes. Monitor the changes. Train staff. Monitor the changes to assure improvement.

The federal regulations do not specify a specific method for quality assessment and assurance. However, the system used must identify when problems exist and provide a way to correct the problems identified, thereby improving quality of care.

Review resident outcomes with the goal of improving care. Selection of issues to be studied in QAA should be made from objective data that measures outcomes of care. Research and use of best practices to improve outcomes. Best practices are proven methods to assure quality care. Revise facility policies and procedures and train staff to do it right the first time. Re-evaluate outcome measurements and use recognized benchmarks to assess progress.

Facility quality indicators are calculated from MDS data sent to the State data base. Start with the CMS Quality Indicators to identify if a problem exists. The Facility Quality Indicator Report includes the facility's data and also include a benchmark percentile to measure against all other facilities in the State.

Resident and family satisfaction questionnaires are another way to identify problem areas. Use the resident and family councils as opportunities to gather information about resident and family concerns. Or ask families and residents to fill out a questionnaire at the time of discharge or annually to gather information about care.

STEPS IN A QAA PROGRAM

1. Assign responsibility for QAA monitoring.

2. Identify the departments to be involved.

3. Target aspects of care to be studied.

4. Develop objective measurements of the quality of care.

5. Establish thresholds for action.

6. Collect data.

7. Evaluate the information collected.

8. Take actions to correct problems identified.

9. Determine whether corrective action was successful.

10. Communicate actions to the governing body.

Overall responsibility for QAA is assigned to a person within the facility designated as the Quality Assessment and Assurance Coordinator. This person's role is to assist each department to identify which aspects of care need to be monitored. The QAA Coordinator may help with development of clinical indicators, data collection and implementation of actions for correction.

C.   Quality Indicators

Quality indicators are measurements that test the outcomes of the activity program. By using measurement devices, such as quality indicators, actual current practice in the facility can be described. The current practices are then evaluated and matched against expectations to identify problems areas that need improvement.

1.   Types of Quality Indicators

There are various ways to look at outcomes of the activity program: Services, Resident Satisfaction, Regulations, Utilization of Services, Management and Cost Analysis (Financial). Actual performance is measured against the quality indicator selected. The clinical indicators will identify the quality of the activity program.

TYPES AND EXAMPLES OF QUALITY INDICATORS

Services   Evaluation of services provided

Number of residents of residents with little or no activity participation

Resident Satisfaction   Resident's perception of service

Resident and Family Questionnaires will be good or excellent

Regulatory   Legal requirements

100% of residents will have a copy of the current activity calendar in their room

Utilization   Volume of services

75% of residents will attend an activity program 3 times a week

Management   Productivity standards

A minimum of 3 one-hour activity programs will be scheduled on weekends

Financial   Cost analysis

Increase intergenerational programs to one each month by adding at least two more kindergarten through second grade volunteer participation annually

Appropriate management of residents with difficult behavioral results in a better living environment for all resident and a more desirable work place for staff

<u>Services</u>	Do the programs offered meet the needs of the current residents in the facility?
<u>Resident Satisfaction</u>	Are the residents happy with the programs or are there other programs that the resident's want that are not now available?
<u>Regulations</u>	Are federal regulations for activity services being met?
<u>Utilization of Services</u>	Does the activity program have enough programs at convenient times of the day and week to meet all residents' needs?
<u>Management</u>	Are residents transported to programs in a timely manner?
<u>Cost Analysis</u>	What is the cost of the programs to the facility?

2.   Methods of Measuring Quality

Quality indicators can be measured by several methods. Measurement is done by observing, interviewing, auditing or collecting data about the actual level of performance. All or any combination of these methods may be part of an effective QAA program.

Some methods of measuring quality are:

- Statistical process control,

- Resident/Family Satisfaction Questionnaires,

- Suggestions Boxes, and

- Self evaluation checklists.

When the actual performance or outcome of the activity program is below expectations, investigation of the reasons and areas for improvement are identified. Plans to change or improve performance and outcome are developed. Actions to correct the problem identified are begun.

Improvement plans can include:

- staff training,

- both inservice and continuing education,

- purchase or repair of equipment,

- reorganization of work flow, and/or

- revisions to policies and procedures.

Once an action plan has been completed, the results of the actions are then re-evaluated to determine actual performance according to the quality indicator. Do a follow up study to check that actions have resulted in quality improvement.

3. Examples of Quality Indicators and Thresholds

The federal government included in the survey process quality indicators based on MDS data that have been transmitted to CMS. These measurements allow surveyors to focus on target areas. Be sure that the data in MDS Item N2 matches CMS's definition (see Chapter 5 Assessment).

Domain 10: Quality of Life

Prevalence of little or no activity [N2 = 2,3]

Each quality indicator contains a measurement of a process or outcome of care and a threshold for action. The threshold for action is expressed by a *number of times* a specific outcome should occur or by a *percentage of times* that an outcome should be achieved.

**EXAMPLES OF CLINICAL INDICATORS
WITH THRESHOLDS FOR ACTION**

- Attendance at (specific) activity program should not be less than (number) of residents.

- Monthly there will be (number) of excursions outside the nursing facility for ambulatory residents.

- Monthly there will be (number) of excursions outside the nursing facility for Non-ambulatory residents.

- Community groups will visit residents (specify number) times a week.

- Residents who do not or cannot attend group activities will have in-room visits daily.

- Positive responses (good or excellent) on Resident Satisfaction Questionnaire will be above 90%.

- Activities occur as scheduled on the activity calendar 90% of the time unless a notice of change has been posted 24 hours prior to the change.

- Responses to recommendations of Resident or Family Council are completed and returned back to the council within three weeks of each meeting.

Quality Indicator   Objective and measurable statements of outcomes of care, staff performance or resident response.

Threshold for Action   The level or point at which care should be evaluated to determine if there is an actual problem or opportunity to improve resident care.

To achieve quality improvement, the QAA committee must carefully study and identify the reasons that the quality indicator was not met.

Identification of possible causes needs to include:

- evaluation of the results of the monitoring and

- drawing appropriate conclusions that will lead to improvement.

Before changing policies or procedures or implementing corrective action, be sure that the correct causal factors have been identified. This may be done by trial or pilot projects on a limited scale to determine the effectiveness of the actions taken.

D. Data Collection

Once quality indicators have been agreed upon, the actual delivery of care is monitored. Additional paperwork is not always necessary. Data can be collected from flow sheets already available, such as, activity attendance records, one to one visit records or computer generated reports based on MDS data.

Checklists may be used for specific monitoring topics:

- resident/family satisfaction surveys,

- review of environmental needs of activity program,

- audit of the activity calendar,

- chart audit for required documentation, and

- minutes of resident or family council meetings.

Case review for residents with special needs such as hearing and vision impairment, or language problems can be used to evaluate the prevalence of such cases or for tracking types of interventions that are most successful.

QUALITY ASSURANCE MONITORING TOOL

Resident Satisfaction Questionnaire   Date:_____

Purpose: To evaluate the resident's satisfaction with the activity program.

QUESTION	RESPONSE
1. Does the activity program meet your interests?	
2. Are there activities that interest you that are not available?	
3. Are you satisfied with the times activities are offered?	
4. Are you satisfied with the number of activities offered?	
5. Are you satisfied with the use of community resources?	
6. Is adequate assistance provided so that you can participate in programs?	
7. Does the activity program address your special needs?	

OTHER REMARKS:

RESIDENT NAME:_____

INTERVIEWED BY_____

QUALITY ASSESSMENT AND ASSURANCE ACTIVITY PROGRAM ENVIRONMENTAL AUDIT TOOL			
Date of Audit_____ Auditor_____			
INDICATORS	**YES**	**NO**	**N/A**
1. Activity Calendar:			
a. Current activities calendar is posted in areas accessible to all resident and staff on each unit			
b. Activity calendar is easy to read and offers a variety of programs			
c. All activities calendars are retained for one year			
2. Program Design: a. Activity programs are provided seven (7) days a week			
b. Evening activities programs are provided once a week			
c. Residents unable to attend programs held in the activity area receive 1:1 contact at least once daily			
3. Activities Area: a. Sufficient space provided in activities area to accommodate scheduled activities without restricting movement and/or active participation of residents			
b. Furnishings are in good repair, clean and at the proper height for activities			
c. Areas are clean and maintained			
d. Area is free of any electrical and other safety haz-			
e. There is adequate lighting/ ventilation			
f. Lavatory is accessible to residents			
g. Temperature maintained at comfort level			
4. Other: a. Transportation of residents to/from programs is provided in a safe, organized, and timely manner			
b. Resident;s schedules (meals, meds, rehab therapy) coordinated with the activity calendar			
Comment on all "NO" answers: Corrective action taken/follow up needed:			

Other useful QAA monitoring tools are resident satisfaction surveys. A positive outcome of care is that the resident is satisfied with the services provided. Resident questionnaires can be completed, individually, by interview, or in a group setting.

Discussion from family and resident council meetings is an excellent source of issues and problems for quality assurance monitoring. Resident and family satisfaction or frequency of complaints is a measurement of quality.

The customer is always right. This motto has special meaning particularly during the survey process. Surveyors are instructed to interview residents and family about the care provided at the facility. Complaints voiced during such interviews will be thoroughly investigated. An ongoing program of interviewing residents and families is an effective means of identifying problems, many that can be quickly and effortlessly resolved.

Suggestion boxes are sometimes used to collect input from staff or family who are not actively participating in any formal means of communicating their ideas. Also designating a Quality Assurance Month with activities and celebrations of QAA accomplishments can increase awareness of the program among staff and stimulate success.

E. Activity Calendar Audit

Evaluation of the activity calendar to assure that it matches with the current resident case-mix is a logical starting point for QAA of Activity Programs. The residents currently in the facility should be reviewed to determine their unique needs. Start by categorizing residents according to their needs and preferences.

Cognition, intact or deficit
Visions Problems
Communication Barriers
Hearing Difficulties
Language other than English

Customary routines such as
    Goes outside at least 1x weekly
    Tobacco use
    Distinct food preferences
    Cultural identification
    Religious participation
    Daily contact with friends/relatives
    Animal companions

Compile a profile of current residents based on their unique needs. Then review the current activity calendar to determine how many hours are offered weekly of activities suitable to resident's needs or customary routines and cultural/religious preferences.

QUALITY ASSESSMENT AND ASSURANCE

ACTIVITY PROGRAM   RESIDENTS NEEDS AUDIT TOOL

Date of Audit_____   Auditor_____

INSTRUCTIONS: List all residents by name and room number. In each column indicate with a check mark any of the resident's special needs or preferences.

Resident Name Room Number	Cognition		Impaired		Non-English Language		Religion/Cultural Preferences	
	Intact	Deficit	Sight	Hearing	Spanish	Other	Catholic	Jewish
Totals								

QUALITY ASSESSMENT AND ASSURANCE

ACTIVITY PROGRAM　　　　　　　RESIDENTS NEEDS AUDIT TOOL

Date of Audit_____　　　Auditor_____

INSTRUCTIONS:　List all activities in the first column. For each scheduled activity identify the number of hours each week that the activity is scheduled and list under as many headings as apply to that activity program.

Title of Activity Program	Cognition		Impaired		Non-English Language		Religion/Cultural Preferences	
	Intact	Deficit	Sight	Hearing	Spanish	Other	Catholic	Jewish
Total hours per week								

QUALITY ASSESSMENT AND ASSURANCE			
ACTIVITY PROGRAM CHART AUDIT TOOL			
NO____RESIDENT NAME_____ROOM_____			

INDICATORS	YES	NO	N/A
1. Assessment:			
a. Completed within 7 days of admission			
b. Content includes			
current and past interests			
physical needs and abilities			
mental needs and abilities			
2. Interdisciplinary Care Plan: Completed on admission for welcome/orientation			
Comprehensive care plan addresses activities needs			
Identifies measurable objective goals			
Plan updated: a. quarterly			
b. modified as needed			
3. Progress Notes: Written at least quarterly			
Assess progress or regress to goals identified in care plan			

COMMENTS:

Dated:_____ Audited by:_____

Copies of activity calendars can be provided to each resident. Those programs that are suitable for the resident can be highlight. This will assure that the resident and family are aware of those activities that the resident prefers or that will benefit the resident. The individualized calendar can also be used to make staff aware of those activities that the resident wishes to attend. Staff can remind the resident to attend or assist the resident by transporting him or her to those activities that are appropriate.

F. Audit Checklists

Checklists are a self-evaluation process. Checklist audits should be done on a regular schedule to identify problems as early as possible. Auditing will not correct a problem but auditing will describe what the problem is. Auditing, however, must have follow up. Identify those persons responsible for correcting an identified deficiency. Verify that deficiencies are corrected.

G. Corrective Action

Quality indicators that are not met alert staff that care should be evaluated to determine if there is an actual problem or opportunity to improve resident care. Unmet indicators do not always mean that quality of care is below standard. Further review of the actual activity program is required to determine the cause of declining attendance.

For example, a clinical indicator could be that at least ten (10) residents are present at the current events program every morning.

- The clinical indicator is the attendance of residents at the current events program.

- The threshold for action is that at least ten (10) residents should attend.

If the month's attendance is 15 or more residents, the clinical indicator is met. If, however, after several months, or during the month of December only, the attendance drops to below ten residents each morning, the quality indicator alerts the staff that something has changed.

Of course, the finding that attendance of an activity program has declined does not necessarily mean that it is a poor quality program. The reason for the change in attendance needs to be investigated and the cause identified. Only when the causal factors are identified can effective corrective action be accomplished. The threshold is an *alert* that something has changed.

For example, some causes after investigation might be:

Two new nursing assistants were recently hired and are slow to bathe and dress residents in the morning delaying their leaving their rooms in time for the current events program.

Review of the types of residents that are in the nursing facility show a change to a larger number of bedfast residents, so that there are no longer ten (10) residents available for whom this program would be suitable.

During the month of December a special Holiday Arts and Craft volunteer conducts a class at the same time as the current events.

After determining the cause for the quality indicator not being met, actions are taken to correct the problem. For example:

Nursing assistants' work load is evaluated by the Director of Nurses and adjustment made so that residents who wish to attend the current events program receive morning care first or early enough to attend the program.

Since there are no longer ten (10) residents who are able to attend the current events program, the clinical indicator can be adjusted to a lower number to reflect the actual needs of the resident population. Additionally, the activity program calendar is re-evaluated to develop programs that would meet the needs of the current residents, such as more in-room programs for bedfast residents.

No changes are indicated in the program, since the Holiday Arts and Crafts was a once a year program by a volunteer. If necessary, a change in time of the current events program for the month of December would allow the residents who attend the arts and crafts to also attend the current events.

H. Follow up of Actions Taken

Summary reports of the QAA process must include problems identified, assessment of causes, corrective actions planned, results of interventions and a re-evaluation of current performance.

Narrative summary reports should be completed by department staff or the QAA Coordinator to track issues identified by the quality assessment and assurance process. The time and effort in assessing practice must be followed with actions taken to improve performance. The documentation should track the problems identified, actions taken, and follow up.

QUALITY ASSESSMENT AND ASSURANCE COMMITTEE

SUMMARY REPORT OF CORRECTIVE ACTIONS

For Meeting of_____

PROBLEMS	ACTION	RESOLUTION

Date_____ Submitted by_____

EXAMPLES OF ACTION FOLLOW UP

PROBLEMS	ACTION	RESOLUTION
Decline in attendance at 10:00 a.m. current events program month of December only	Conflicts with Holiday Arts and Crafts, change to 4:00 p.m. for December only.	December attendance back to 10 to 15 residents now that time has changed
Activity program calendar changed 5 times this month	Last minute changes for Christmas Singers to avoid conflicts	Confirm as many as possible (75%) of special Christmas visits with outside volunteers before Thanksgiving

I.   Departmental Preparation

Quality assessment and assurance applies to every department in the nursing facility. Desired outcomes of care are identified. Clinical indicators which measure actual practice are developed and/or approved by each department. If QAA is to work, staff participation is essential. Staff must agree to the standards against which their services will be measured.

All departments report quarterly to the Quality Assessment and Assurance Committee about their monitoring activities. These reports are made a part of the QAA minutes with copies to the administrator.

Quarterly reports summarize the monitoring activities:

- the problems identified

- the investigation of the causes

- the corrective action taken.

QUALITY ASSESSMENT AND ASSURANCE REPORT

DEPARTMENT: Activity Program   For the months of _____

QUALITY INDICATORS

1.   Ambulatory residents will have weekly excursions outside facility.

2.   Non-ambulatory residents will have monthly excursions outside facility.

3.   Volunteer groups from the community will be scheduled for visits twice a week.

4.   At least fifteen (15) residents will attend Resident Council.

MONTHS OF			
Number of excursions outside facility for:			
Ambulatory residents			
Non-ambulatory residents			
Attendance at Resident Council (Number of Attendees)			
Number of visits from community groups			
Religious			
Intergenerational			
Special therapy			
Other:			
Number of residents with 1:1 visits			
By Volunteers			
By activity program staff			

COMMENTS:

Dated_____Submitted By_____

QUALITY ASSESSMENT AND ASSURANCE REPORT

DEPARTMENT: Activity Program   For the Month of:_____

Problems identified by Audit Tools_____

_____

_____

_____

_____

Problems identified at Resident Satisfaction Surveys_____

_____

_____

_____

Problems identified in Resident or Family Council_____

_____

_____

_____

_____

New Policy and Procedures_____

_____

_____

Dated_____ Submitted by_____

Appendix

Numeric Identifier_____

MINIMUM DATA SET (MDS) — *VERSION 2.0*
FOR NURSING HOME RESIDENT ASSESSMENT AND CARE SCREENING

BASIC ASSESSMENT TRACKING FORM

SECTION AA. IDENTIFICATION INFORMATION

1.	RESIDENT NAME⊚				
		a. (First)	b. (Middle Initial)	c. (Last)	d. (Jr/Sr)

2.	GENDER⊚	1. Male	2. Female

3.	BIRTHDATE⊚	☐☐ — ☐☐ — ☐☐☐☐
		Month Day Year

4.	RACE/⊚ ETHNICITY	1. American Indian/Alaskan Native 4. Hispanic 2. Asian/Pacific Islander 5. White, not of 3. Black, not of Hispanic origin Hispanic origin

5.	SOCIAL SECURITY⊚ AND MEDICARE NUMBERS⊚ [C in 1st box if non med. no.]	a. Social Security Number ☐☐☐—☐☐—☐☐☐☐ b. Medicare number (or comparable railroad insurance number)

6.	FACILITY PROVIDER NO.⊚	a. State No. b. Federal No.

7.	MEDICAID NO. ["+" if pending, "N" if not a Medicaid recipient] ⊚	

8.	REASONS FOR ASSESSMENT	[Note—Other codes do not apply to this form]
		a. Primary reason for assessment
		  1. Admission assessment (required by day 14)
		  2. Annual assessment
		  3. Significant change in status assessment
		  4. Significant correction of prior full assessment
		  5. Quarterly review assessment
		  10. Significant correction of prior quarterly assessment
		  0. *NONE OF ABOVE*
		b. *Codes for assessments required for Medicare PPS or the State*
		  1. *Medicare 5 day assessment*
		  2. *Medicare 30 day assessment*
		  3. *Medicare 60 day assessment*
		  4. *Medicare 90 day assessment*
		  5. *Medicare readmission/return assessment*
		  6. *Other state required assessment*
		  7. *Medicare 14 day assessment*
		  8. *Other Medicare required assessment*

9. Signatures of Persons who Completed a Portion of the Accompanying Assessment or Tracking Form

I certify that the accompanying information accurately reflects resident assessment or tracking information for this resident and that I collected or coordinated collection of this information on the dates specified. To the best of my knowledge, this information was collected in accordance with applicable Medicare and Medicaid requirements. I understand that this information is used as a basis for ensuring that residents receive appropriate and quality care, and as a basis for payment from federal funds. I further understand that payment of such federal funds and continued participation in the government-funded health care programs is conditioned on the accuracy and truthfulness of this information, and that I may be personally subject to or may subject my organization to substantial criminal, civil, and/or administrative penalties for submitting false information. I also certify that I am authorized to submit this information by this facility on its behalf.

Signature and Title	Sections	Date
a.		
b.		
c.		
d.		
e.		
f.		
g.		
h.		
i.		
j.		
k.		
l.		

GENERAL INSTRUCTIONS

Complete this information for submission with all full and quarterly assessments (Admission, Annual, Significant Change, State or Medicare required assessments, or Quarterly Reviews, etc.)

⊚ = Key items for computerized resident tracking

☐ = When box blank, must enter number or letter   [a.] = When letter in box, check if condition applies

MDS 2.0 September, 2000

Resident _____ Numeric Identifier _____

MINIMUM DATA SET (MDS) — *VERSION 2.0*
FOR NURSING HOME RESIDENT ASSESSMENT AND CARE SCREENING

BACKGROUND (FACE SHEET) INFORMATION AT ADMISSION

SECTION AB. DEMOGRAPHIC INFORMATION

1.	DATE OF ENTRY	Date the stay began. Note — Does not include readmission if record was closed at time of temporary discharge to hospital, etc. In such cases, use prior admission date Month — Day — Year
2.	ADMITTED FROM (AT ENTRY)	1. Private home/apt. with no home health services 2. Private home/apt. with home health services 3. Board and care/assisted living/group home 4. Nursing home 5. Acute care hospital 6. Psychiatric hospital, MR/DD facility 7. Rehabilitation hospital 8. Other
3.	LIVED ALONE (PRIOR TO ENTRY)	0. No 1. Yes 2. In other facility
4.	ZIP CODE OF PRIOR PRIMARY RESIDENCE	
5.	RESIDENTIAL HISTORY 5 YEARS PRIOR TO ENTRY	(Check all settings resident lived in during 5 years prior to date of entry given in item AB1 above) Prior stay at this nursing home — a. Stay in other nursing home — b. Other residential facility—board and care home, assisted living, group home — c. MH/psychiatric setting — d. MR/DD setting — e. NONE OF ABOVE — f.
6.	LIFETIME OCCUPA-TION(S) [Put "/" between two occupations]	
7.	EDUCATION (Highest Level Completed)	1. No schooling 5. Technical or trade school 2. 8th grade/less 6. Some college 3. 9-11 grades 7. Bachelor's degree 4. High school 8. Graduate degree
8.	LANGUAGE	(Code for correct response) a. Primary Language 0. English 1. Spanish 2. French 3. Other b. If other, specify
9.	MENTAL HEALTH HISTORY	Does resident's RECORD indicate any history of mental retardation, mental illness, or developmental disability problem? 0. No 1. Yes
10.	CONDITIONS RELATED TO MR/DD STATUS	(Check all conditions that are related to MR/DD status that were manifested before age 22, and are likely to continue indefinitely) Not applicable—no MR/DD (Skip to AB11) — a. MR/DD with organic condition Down's syndrome — b. Autism — c. Epilepsy — d. Other organic condition related to MR/DD — e. MR/DD with no organic condition — f.
11.	DATE BACK-GROUND INFORMA-TION COMPLETED	Month — Day — Year

SECTION AC. CUSTOMARY ROUTINE

1.	CUSTOMARY ROUTINE (In year prior to DATE OF ENTRY to this nursing home, or year last in community if now being admitted from another nursing home)	(Check all that apply. If all information UNKNOWN, check last box only.)	
		CYCLE OF DAILY EVENTS	
		Stays up late at night (e.g., after 9 pm)	a.
		Naps regularly during day (at least 1 hour)	b.
		Goes out 1+ days a week	c.
		Stays busy with hobbies, reading, or fixed daily routine	d.
		Spends most of time alone or watching TV	e.
		Moves independently indoors (with appliances, if used)	f.
		Use of tobacco products at least daily	g.
		NONE OF ABOVE	h.
		EATING PATTERNS	
		Distinct food preferences	i.
		Eats between meals all or most days	j.
		Use of alcoholic beverage(s) at least weekly	k.
		NONE OF ABOVE	l.
		ADL PATTERNS	
		In bedclothes much of day	m.
		Wakens to toilet all or most nights	n.
		Has irregular bowel movement pattern	o.
		Showers for bathing	p.
		Bathing in PM	q.
		NONE OF ABOVE	r.
		INVOLVEMENT PATTERNS	
		Daily contact with relatives/close friends	s.
		Usually attends church, temple, synagogue (etc.)	t.
		Finds strength in faith	u.
		Daily animal companion/presence	v.
		Involved in group activities	w.
		NONE OF ABOVE	x.
		UNKNOWN—Resident/family unable to provide information	y.

SECTION AD. FACE SHEET SIGNATURES

SIGNATURES OF PERSONS COMPLETING FACE SHEET:

a. Signature of RN Assessment Coordinator   Date

I certify that the accompanying information accurately reflects resident assessment or tracking information for this resident and that I collected or coordinated collection of this information on the dates specified. To the best of my knowledge, this information was collected in accordance with applicable Medicare and Medicaid requirements. I understand that this information is used as a basis for ensuring that residents receive appropriate and quality care, and as a basis for payment from federal funds. I further understand that payment of such federal funds and continued participation in the government-funded health care programs is conditioned on the accuracy and truthfulness of this information, and that I may be personally subject to or may subject my organization to substantial criminal, civil, and/or administrative penalties for submitting false information. I also certify that I am authorized to submit this information by this facility on its behalf.

Signature and Title	Sections	Date
b.		
c.		
d.		
e.		
f.		
g.		

☐ = When box blank, must enter number or letter   ☐a. = When letter in box, check if condition applies

MDS 2.0 September, 2000

Resident _____   Numeric Identifier _____

MINIMUM DATA SET (MDS) — *VERSION 2.0*
FOR NURSING HOME RESIDENT ASSESSMENT AND CARE SCREENING
FULL ASSESSMENT FORM
(Status in last 7 days, unless other time frame indicated)

SECTION A. IDENTIFICATION AND BACKGROUND INFORMATION

1.	RESIDENT NAME				
		a. (First)	b. (Middle initial)	c. (Last)	d. (Jr/Sr)

2.	ROOM NUMBER	☐☐☐☐☐

3. ASSESSMENT REFERENCE DATE
a. Last day of MDS observation period
☐☐ — ☐☐ — ☐☐☐☐
Month Day Year
b. Original (0) or corrected copy of form (enter number of correction) ☐

4a. DATE OF REENTRY Date of reentry from most recent temporary discharge to a hospital in last 90 days (or since last assessment or admission if less than 90 days)
☐☐ — ☐☐ — ☐☐☐☐
Month Day Year

5. MARITAL STATUS
1. Never married 3. Widowed 5. Divorced
2. Married 4. Separated ☐

6. MEDICAL RECORD NO. ☐☐☐☐☐☐☐☐☐☐

7. CURRENT PAYMENT SOURCES FOR N.H. STAY *(Billing Office to indicate; check all that apply in last 30 days)*
Medicaid per diem	a.	VA per diem		f.
Medicare per diem	b.	Self or family pays for full per diem		g.
Medicaid ancillary part A	c.	Medicaid resident liability or Medicare co-payment		h.
Medicare ancillary part B	d.	Private insurance per diem (including co-payment)		i.
CHAMPUS per diem	e.	Other per diem		j.

8. REASONS FOR ASSESSMENT
[Note—If this is a discharge or reentry assessment, only a limited subset of MDS items need be completed]
a. Primary reason for assessment
1. Admission assessment (required by day 14)
2. Annual assessment
3. Significant change in status assessment
4. Significant correction of prior full assessment
5. Quarterly review assessment
6. Discharged—return not anticipated
7. Discharged—return anticipated
8. Discharged prior to completing initial assessment
9. Reentry
10. Significant correction of prior quarterly assessment
0. *NONE OF ABOVE*

b. Codes for assessments required for Medicare PPS or the State
1. Medicare 5 day assessment
2. Medicare 30 day assessment
3. Medicare 60 day assessment
4. Medicare 90 day assessment
5. Medicare readmission/return assessment
6. Other state required assessment
7. Medicare 14 day assessment
8. Other Medicare required assessment

9. RESPONSIBILITY/ LEGAL GUARDIAN *(Check all that apply)*
Legal guardian	a.	Durable power attorney/financial	d.
Other legal oversight	b.	Family member responsible	e.
Durable power of attorney/health care	c.	Patient responsible for self	f.
		NONE OF ABOVE	g.

10. ADVANCED DIRECTIVES *(For those items with supporting documentation in the medical record, check all that apply)*
Living will	a.	Feeding restrictions	f.
Do not resuscitate	b.	Medication restrictions	g.
Do not hospitalize	c.	Other treatment restrictions	h.
Organ donation	d.		
Autopsy request	e.	NONE OF ABOVE	i.

SECTION B. COGNITIVE PATTERNS

1.	COMATOSE	*(Persistent vegetative state/no discernible consciousness)*	
		0. No 1. Yes (If yes, skip to Section G)	

2. MEMORY *(Recall of what was learned or known)*
a. Short-term memory OK—seems/appears to recall after 5 minutes
0. Memory OK 1. Memory problem
b. Long-term memory OK—seems/appears to recall long past
0. Memory OK 1. Memory problem

3. MEMORY/ RECALL ABILITY *(Check all that resident was normally able to recall during last 7 days)*
Current season	a.	That he/she is in a nursing home	d.
Location of own room	b.		
Staff names/faces	c.	NONE OF ABOVE are recalled	e.

4. COGNITIVE SKILLS FOR DAILY DECISION-MAKING *(Made decisions regarding tasks of daily life)*
0. INDEPENDENT—decisions consistent/reasonable
1. MODIFIED INDEPENDENCE—some difficulty in new situations only
2. MODERATELY IMPAIRED—decisions poor; cues/supervision required
3. SEVERELY IMPAIRED—never/rarely made decisions

5. INDICATORS OF DELIRIUM— PERIODIC DISORDERED THINKING/ AWARENESS *(Code for behavior in the last 7 days.) [Note: Accurate assessment requires conversations with staff and family who have direct knowledge of resident's behavior over this time].*
0. Behavior not present
1. Behavior present, not of recent onset
2. Behavior present, over last 7 days appears different from resident's usual functioning (e.g., new onset or worsening)

a. EASILY DISTRACTED—(e.g., difficulty paying attention; gets sidetracked)
b. PERIODS OF ALTERED PERCEPTION OR AWARENESS OF SURROUNDINGS—(e.g., moves lips or talks to someone not present; believes he/she is somewhere else; confuses night and day)
c. EPISODES OF DISORGANIZED SPEECH—(e.g., speech is incoherent, nonsensical, irrelevant, or rambling from subject to subject; loses train of thought)
d. PERIODS OF RESTLESSNESS—(e.g., fidgeting or picking at skin, clothing, napkins, etc; frequent position changes; repetitive physical movements or calling out)
e. PERIODS OF LETHARGY—(e.g., sluggishness; staring into space; difficult to arouse; little body movement)
f. MENTAL FUNCTION VARIES OVER THE COURSE OF THE DAY—(e.g., sometimes better, sometimes worse; behaviors sometimes present, sometimes not)

6. CHANGE IN COGNITIVE STATUS Resident's cognitive status, skills, or abilities have changed as compared to status of 90 days ago (or since last assessment if less than 90 days)
0. No change 1. Improved 2. Deteriorated

SECTION C. COMMUNICATION/HEARING PATTERNS

1. HEARING *(With hearing appliance, if used)*
0. HEARS ADEQUATELY—normal talk, TV, phone
1. MINIMAL DIFFICULTY when not in quiet setting
2. HEARS IN SPECIAL SITUATIONS ONLY—speaker has to adjust tonal quality and speak distinctly
3. HIGHLY IMPAIRED/absence of useful hearing

2. COMMUNICATION DEVICES/ TECHNIQUES *(Check all that apply during last 7 days)*
Hearing aid, present and used	a.
Hearing aid, present and not used regularly	b.
Other receptive comm. techniques used (e.g., lip reading)	c.
NONE OF ABOVE	d.

3. MODES OF EXPRESSION *(Check all used by resident to make needs known)*
Speech	a.	Signs/gestures/sounds	d.
Writing messages to express or clarify needs	b.	Communication board	e.
American sign language or Braille	c.	Other	f.
		NONE OF ABOVE	g.

4. MAKING SELF UNDERSTOOD *(Expressing information content—however able)*
0. UNDERSTOOD
1. USUALLY UNDERSTOOD—difficulty finding words or finishing thoughts
2. SOMETIMES UNDERSTOOD—ability is limited to making concrete requests
3. RARELY/NEVER UNDERSTOOD

5. SPEECH CLARITY *(Code for speech in the last 7 days)*
0. CLEAR SPEECH—distinct, intelligible words
1. UNCLEAR SPEECH—slurred, mumbled words
2. NO SPEECH—absence of spoken words

6. ABILITY TO UNDERSTAND OTHERS *(Understanding verbal information content—however able)*
0. UNDERSTANDS
1. USUALLY UNDERSTANDS—may miss some part/intent of message
2. SOMETIMES UNDERSTANDS—responds adequately to simple, direct communication
3. RARELY/NEVER UNDERSTANDS

7. CHANGE IN COMMUNICATION/ HEARING Resident's ability to express, understand, or hear information has changed as compared to status of 90 days ago (or since last assessment if less than 90 days)
0. No change 1. Improved 2. Deteriorated

☐ = When box blank, must enter number or letter   ☐a. = When letter in box, check if condition applies

MDS 2.0 September, 2000

Appendix

Resident _____ **Numeric Identifier** _____

SECTION D. VISION PATTERNS

1. VISION (Ability to see in adequate light and with glasses if used)
0. ADEQUATE—sees fine detail, including regular print in newspapers/books
1. IMPAIRED—sees large print, but not regular print in newspapers/books
2. MODERATELY IMPAIRED—limited vision; not able to see newspaper headlines, but can identify objects
3. HIGHLY IMPAIRED—object identification in question, but eyes appear to follow objects
4. SEVERELY IMPAIRED—no vision or sees only light, colors, or shapes; eyes do not appear to follow objects

2. VISUAL LIMITATIONS/DIFFICULTIES
a. Side vision problems—decreased peripheral vision (e.g., leaves food on one side of tray, difficulty traveling, bumps into people and objects, misjudges placement of chair when seating self)
b. Experiences any of following: sees halos or rings around lights; sees flashes of light; sees "curtains" over eyes
c. NONE OF ABOVE

3. VISUAL APPLIANCES Glasses; contact lenses; magnifying glass
0. No   1. Yes

SECTION E. MOOD AND BEHAVIOR PATTERNS

1. INDICATORS OF DEPRESSION, ANXIETY, SAD MOOD (Code for indicators observed in last 30 days, irrespective of the assumed cause)
0. Indicator not exhibited in last 30 days
1. Indicator of this type exhibited up to five days a week
2. Indicator of this type exhibited daily or almost daily (6, 7 days a week)

VERBAL EXPRESSIONS OF DISTRESS
a. Resident made negative statements—e.g., "Nothing matters; Would rather be dead; What's the use; Regrets having lived so long; Let me die"
b. Repetitive questions—e.g., "Where do I go; What do I do?"
c. Repetitive verbalizations—e.g., calling out for help, ("God help me")
d. Persistent anger with self or others—e.g., easily annoyed, anger at placement in nursing home; anger at care received
e. Self deprecation—e.g., "I am nothing; I am of no use to anyone"
f. Expressions of what appear to be unrealistic fears—e.g., fear of being abandoned, left alone, being with others
g. Recurrent statements that something terrible is about to happen—e.g., believes he or she is about to die, have a heart attack

h. Repetitive health complaints—e.g., persistently seeks medical attention, obsessive concern with body functions
i. Repetitive anxious complaints/concerns (non-health related) e.g., persistently seeks attention/reassurance regarding schedules, meals, laundry, clothing, relationship issues

SLEEP-CYCLE ISSUES
j. Unpleasant mood in morning
k. Insomnia/change in usual sleep pattern

SAD, APATHETIC, ANXIOUS APPEARANCE
l. Sad, pained, worried facial expressions—e.g., furrowed brows
m. Crying, tearfulness
n. Repetitive physical movements—e.g., pacing, hand wringing, restlessness, fidgeting, picking

LOSS OF INTEREST
o. Withdrawal from activities of interest—e.g., no interest in long standing activities or being with family/friends
p. Reduced social interaction

2. MOOD PERSISTENCE One or more indicators of depressed, sad or anxious mood were not easily altered by attempts to "cheer up", console, or reassure the resident over last 7 days
0. No mood indicators   1. Indicators present, easily altered   2. Indicators present, not easily altered

3. CHANGE IN MOOD Resident's mood status has changed as compared to status of 90 days ago (or since last assessment if less than 90 days)
0. No change   1. Improved   2. Deteriorated

4. BEHAVIORAL SYMPTOMS
(A) Behavioral symptom frequency in last 7 days
0. Behavior not exhibited in last 7 days
1. Behavior of this type occurred 1 to 3 days in last 7 days
2. Behavior of this type occurred 4 to 6 days, but less than daily
3. Behavior of this type occurred daily

(B) Behavioral symptom alterability in last 7 days
0. Behavior not present OR behavior was easily altered
1. Behavior was not easily altered

a. WANDERING (moved with no rational purpose, seemingly oblivious to needs or safety)
b. VERBALLY ABUSIVE BEHAVIORAL SYMPTOMS (others were threatened, screamed at, cursed at)
c. PHYSICALLY ABUSIVE BEHAVIORAL SYMPTOMS (others were hit, shoved, scratched, sexually abused)
d. SOCIALLY INAPPROPRIATE/DISRUPTIVE BEHAVIORAL SYMPTOMS (made disruptive sounds, noisiness, screaming, self-abusive acts, sexual behavior or disrobing in public, smeared/threw food/feces, hoarding, rummaged through others' belongings)
e. RESISTS CARE (resisted taking medications/injections, ADL assistance, or eating)

5. CHANGE IN BEHAVIORAL SYMPTOMS Resident's behavior status has changed as compared to status of 90 days ago (or since last assessment if less than 90 days)
0. No change   1. Improved   2. Deteriorated

SECTION F. PSYCHOSOCIAL WELL-BEING

1. SENSE OF INITIATIVE/INVOLVEMENT
a. At ease interacting with others
b. At ease doing planned or structured activities
c. At ease doing self-initiated activities
d. Establishes own goals
f. Pursues involvement in life of facility (e.g., makes/keeps friends; involved in group activities; responds positively to new activities; assists at religious services)
g. Accepts invitations into most group activities
NONE OF ABOVE

2. UNSETTLED RELATIONSHIPS
a. Covert/open conflict with or repeated criticism of staff
b. Unhappy with roommate
c. Unhappy with residents other than roommate
d. Openly expresses conflict/anger with family/friends
e. Absence of personal contact with family/friends
f. Recent loss of close family member/friend
g. Does not adjust easily to change in routines
h. NONE OF ABOVE

3. PAST ROLES
a. Strong identification with past roles and life status
b. Expresses sadness/anger/empty feeling over lost roles/status
c. Resident perceives that daily routine (customary routine, activities) is very different from prior pattern in the community
NONE OF ABOVE

SECTION G. PHYSICAL FUNCTIONING AND STRUCTURAL PROBLEMS

1. (A) ADL SELF-PERFORMANCE—(Code for resident's PERFORMANCE OVER ALL SHIFTS during last 7 days—Not including setup)
0. INDEPENDENT—No help or oversight —OR— Help/oversight provided only 1 or 2 times during last 7 days
1. SUPERVISION—Oversight, encouragement or cueing provided 3 or more times during last 7 days —OR— Supervision (3 or more times) plus physical assistance provided only 1 or 2 times during last 7 days
2. LIMITED ASSISTANCE—Resident highly involved in activity; received physical help in guided maneuvering of limbs or other nonweight bearing assistance 3 or more times —OR—More help provided only 1 or 2 times during last 7 days
3. EXTENSIVE ASSISTANCE—While resident performed part of activity, over last 7-day period, help of following type(s) provided 3 or more times:
—Weight-bearing support
—Full staff performance during part (but not all) of last 7 days
4. TOTAL DEPENDENCE—Full staff performance of activity during entire 7 days
8. ACTIVITY DID NOT OCCUR during entire 7 days

(B) ADL SUPPORT PROVIDED—(Code for MOST SUPPORT PROVIDED OVER ALL SHIFTS during last 7 days; code regardless of resident's self-performance classification)
0. No setup or physical help from staff
1. Setup help only
2. One person physical assist
3. Two+ persons physical assist
8. ADL activity itself did not occur during entire 7 days

			(A) SELF-PERF	(B) SUPPORT
a.	BED MOBILITY	How resident moves to and from lying position, turns side to side, and positions body while in bed		
b.	TRANSFER	How resident moves between surfaces—to/from: bed, chair, wheelchair, standing position (EXCLUDE to/from bath/toilet)		
c.	WALK IN ROOM	How resident walks between locations in his/her room		
d.	WALK IN CORRIDOR	How resident walks in corridor on unit		
e.	LOCOMOTION ON UNIT	How resident moves between locations in his/her room and adjacent corridor on same floor. If in wheelchair, self-sufficiency once in chair		
f.	LOCOMOTION OFF UNIT	How resident moves to and returns from off unit locations (e.g., areas set aside for dining, activities, or treatments). If facility has only one floor, how resident moves to and from distant areas on the floor. If in wheelchair, self-sufficiency once in chair		
g.	DRESSING	How resident puts on, fastens, and takes off all items of street clothing, including donning/removing prosthesis		
h.	EATING	How resident eats and drinks (regardless of skill). Includes intake of nourishment by other means (e.g., tube feeding, total parenteral nutrition)		
i.	TOILET USE	How resident uses the toilet room (or commode, bedpan, urinal); transfer on/off toilet, cleanses, changes pad, manages ostomy or catheter, adjusts clothes		
j.	PERSONAL HYGIENE	How resident maintains personal hygiene, including combing hair, brushing teeth, shaving, applying makeup, washing/drying face, hands, and perineum (EXCLUDE baths and showers)		

MDS 2.0 September, 2000

Documentation in a SNAP

Resident _____   Numeric Identifier _____

2.	BATHING	How resident takes full-body bath/shower, sponge bath, and transfers in/out of tub/shower (EXCLUDE washing of back and hair.) *Code for most dependent in self-performance and support.* (A) BATHING SELF-PERFORMANCE codes appear below	(A)	(B)
		0. Independent—No help provided		
		1. Supervision—Oversight help only		
		2. Physical help limited to transfer only		
		3. Physical help in part of bathing activity		
		4. Total dependence		
		8. Activity itself did not occur during entire 7 days *(Bathing support codes are as defined in item 1, code B above)*		

3.	TEST FOR BALANCE *(see training manual)*	*(Code for ability during test in the last 7 days)* 0. Maintained position as required in test 1. Unsteady, but able to rebalance self without physical support 2. Partial physical support during test; or stands (sits) but does not follow directions for test 3. Not able to attempt test without physical help	
		a. Balance while standing	
		b. Balance while sitting—position, trunk control	

4.	FUNCTIONAL LIMITATION IN RANGE OF MOTION *(see training manual)*	*(Code for limitations during last 7 days that interfered with daily functions or placed resident at risk of injury)* (A) RANGE OF MOTION (B) VOLUNTARY MOVEMENT 0. No limitation 0. No loss 1. Limitation on one side 1. Partial loss 2. Limitation on both sides 2. Full loss	(A)	(B)
		a. Neck		
		b. Arm—Including shoulder or elbow		
		c. Hand—Including wrist or fingers		
		d. Leg—Including hip or knee		
		e. Foot—Including ankle or toes		
		f. Other limitation or loss		

5.	MODES OF LOCOMOTION	*(Check all that apply during last 7 days)*	
		Cane/walker/crutch a.	Wheelchair primary mode of locomotion d.
		Wheeled self b.	
		Other person wheeled c.	NONE OF ABOVE e.

6.	MODES OF TRANSFER	*(Check all that apply during last 7 days)*	
		Bedfast all or most of time a.	Lifted mechanically d.
		Bed rails used for bed mobility or transfer b.	Transfer aid (e.g., slide board, trapeze, cane, walker, brace) e.
		Lifted manually c.	NONE OF ABOVE f.

7.	TASK SEGMENTATION	Some or all of ADL activities were broken into subtasks during last 7 days so that resident could perform them 0. No 1. Yes	

8.	ADL FUNCTIONAL REHABILITATION POTENTIAL	Resident believes he/she is capable of increased independence in at least some ADLs	a.
		Direct care staff believe resident is capable of increased independence in at least some ADLs	b.
		Resident able to perform tasks/activity but is very slow	c.
		Difference in ADL Self-Performance or ADL Support, comparing mornings to evenings	d.
		NONE OF ABOVE	e.

9.	CHANGE IN ADL FUNCTION	Resident's ADL self-performance status has changed as compared to status of 90 days ago (or since last assessment if less than 90 days) 0. No change 1. Improved 2. Deteriorated	

SECTION H. CONTINENCE IN LAST 14 DAYS

1.	CONTINENCE SELF-CONTROL CATEGORIES *(Code for resident's PERFORMANCE OVER ALL SHIFTS)*
	0. CONTINENT—Complete control *[includes use of indwelling urinary catheter or ostomy device that does not leak urine or stool]*
	1. USUALLY CONTINENT—BLADDER, incontinent episodes once a week or less; BOWEL, less than weekly
	2. OCCASIONALLY INCONTINENT—BLADDER, 2 or more times a week but not daily; BOWEL, once a week
	3. FREQUENTLY INCONTINENT—BLADDER, tended to be incontinent daily, but some control present (e.g., on day shift); BOWEL, 2-3 times a week
	4. INCONTINENT—Had inadequate control BLADDER, multiple daily episodes; BOWEL, all (or almost all) of the time

a.	BOWEL CONTINENCE	Control of bowel movement, with appliance or bowel continence programs, if employed	
b.	BLADDER CONTINENCE	Control of urinary bladder function (if dribbles, volume insufficient to soak through underpants), with appliances (e.g., foley) or continence programs, if employed	

2.	BOWEL ELIMINATION PATTERN	Bowel elimination pattern regular—at least one movement every three days a.	Diarrhea c.
			Fecal impaction d.
		Constipation b.	NONE OF ABOVE e.

MDS 2.0 September, 2000

3.	APPLIANCES AND PROGRAMS	Any scheduled toileting plan a.	Did not use toilet room/commode/urinal f.
		Bladder retraining program b.	Pads/briefs used g.
		External (condom) catheter c.	Enemas/irrigation h.
		Indwelling catheter d.	Ostomy present i.
		Intermittent catheter e.	NONE OF ABOVE

4.	CHANGE IN URINARY CONTINENCE	Resident's urinary continence has changed as compared to status of 90 days ago (or since last assessment if less than 90 days) 0. No change 1. Improved 2. Deteriorated	

SECTION I. DISEASE DIAGNOSES

Check only those diseases that have a relationship to current ADL status, cognitive status, mood and behavior status, medical treatments, nursing monitoring, or risk of death. (Do not list inactive diagnoses.)

1.	DISEASES	*(If none apply, CHECK the NONE OF ABOVE box)*	
		ENDOCRINE/METABOLIC/NUTRITIONAL	Hemiplegia/Hemiparesis v.
			Multiple sclerosis w.
		Diabetes mellitus a.	Paraplegia x.
		Hyperthyroidism b.	Parkinson's disease y.
		Hypothyroidism c.	Quadriplegia z.
		HEART/CIRCULATION	Seizure disorder aa.
		Arteriosclerotic heart disease (ASHD) d.	Transient ischemic attack (TIA) bb.
		Cardiac dysrhythmias e.	Traumatic brain injury cc.
		Congestive heart failure f.	**PSYCHIATRIC/MOOD**
		Deep vein thrombosis g.	Anxiety disorder dd.
		Hypertension h.	Depression ee.
		Hypotension i.	Manic depression (bipolar disease) ff.
		Peripheral vascular disease j.	Schizophrenia gg.
		Other cardiovascular disease k.	**PULMONARY**
		MUSCULOSKELETAL	Asthma hh.
		Arthritis l.	Emphysema/COPD ii.
		Hip fracture m.	**SENSORY**
		Missing limb (e.g., amputation) n.	Cataracts jj.
		Osteoporosis o.	Diabetic retinopathy kk.
		Pathological bone fracture p.	Glaucoma ll.
		NEUROLOGICAL	Macular degeneration mm.
		Alzheimer's disease q.	**OTHER**
		Aphasia r.	Allergies nn.
		Cerebral palsy s.	Anemia oo.
		Cerebrovascular accident (stroke) t.	Cancer pp.
			Renal failure qq.
		Dementia other than Alzheimer's disease u.	NONE OF ABOVE rr.

2.	INFECTIONS	*(If none apply, CHECK the NONE OF ABOVE box)*	
		Antibiotic resistant infection (e.g., Methicillin resistant staph) a.	Septicemia g.
			Sexually transmitted diseases h.
		Clostridium difficile (c. diff.) b.	Tuberculosis i.
		Conjunctivitis c.	Urinary tract infection in last 30 days j.
		HIV infection d.	Viral hepatitis k.
		Pneumonia e.	Wound infection l.
		Respiratory infection f.	NONE OF ABOVE m.

3.	OTHER CURRENT OR MORE DETAILED DIAGNOSES AND ICD-9 CODES	a. _____	⎢ ⎢ ⎢•⎢ ⎢
		b. _____	⎢ ⎢ ⎢•⎢ ⎢
		c. _____	⎢ ⎢ ⎢•⎢ ⎢
		d. _____	⎢ ⎢ ⎢•⎢ ⎢
		e. _____	⎢ ⎢ ⎢•⎢ ⎢

SECTION J. HEALTH CONDITIONS

1.	PROBLEM CONDITIONS	*(Check all problems present in last 7 days unless other time frame is indicated)*	
		INDICATORS OF FLUID STATUS	Dizziness/Vertigo f.
			Edema g.
		Weight gain or loss of 3 or more pounds within a 7 day period a.	Fever h.
			Hallucinations i.
			Internal bleeding j.
		Inability to lie flat due to shortness of breath b.	Recurrent lung aspirations in last 90 days k.
		Dehydrated; output exceeds input c.	Shortness of breath l.
			Syncope (fainting) m.
		Insufficient fluid; did NOT consume all/almost all liquids provided during last 3 days d.	Unsteady gait n.
			Vomiting o.
		OTHER	NONE OF ABOVE p.
		Delusions e.	

Resident _____   Numeric Identifier _____

2.	PAIN SYMPTOMS	(Code the highest level of pain present in the last 7 days)		
		a. FREQUENCY with which resident complains or shows evidence of pain	b. INTENSITY of pain	
		0. No pain (skip to J4)	1. Mild pain	
		1. Pain less than daily	2. Moderate pain	
		2. Pain daily	3. Times when pain is horrible or excruciating	

3.	PAIN SITE	(If pain present, check all sites that apply in last 7 days)		
		Back pain	a.	Incisional pain	f.
		Bone pain		Joint pain (other than hip)	g.
		Chest pain while doing usual activities		Soft tissue pain (e.g., lesion, muscle)	h.
		Headache	d.	Stomach pain	i.
		Hip pain	e.	Other	j.

4.	ACCIDENTS	(Check all that apply)		
		Fell in past 30 days	a.	Hip fracture in last 180 days	c.
		Fell in past 31-180 days	b.	Other fracture in last 180 days	d.
				NONE OF ABOVE	e.

5.	STABILITY OF CONDITIONS	Conditions/diseases make resident's cognitive, ADL, mood or behavior patterns unstable—(fluctuating, precarious, or deteriorating)	a.
		Resident experiencing an acute episode or a flare-up of a recurrent or chronic problem	b.
		End-stage disease, 6 or fewer months to live	c.
		NONE OF ABOVE	d.

SECTION K. ORAL/NUTRITIONAL STATUS

1.	ORAL PROBLEMS	Chewing problem	a.
		Swallowing problem	b.
		Mouth pain	c.
		NONE OF ABOVE	d.

2.	HEIGHT AND WEIGHT	Record (a.) height in inches and (b.) weight in pounds. Base weight on most recent measure in last 30 days; measure weight consistently in accord with standard facility practice—e.g., in a.m. after voiding, before meal, with shoes off, and in nightclothes	
		a. HT (in.)	b. WT (lb.)

3.	WEIGHT CHANGE	a. Weight loss—5 % or more in last 30 days; or 10 % or more in last 180 days	
		0. No 1. Yes	
		b. Weight gain—5 % or more in last 30 days; or 10 % or more in last 180 days	
		0. No 1. Yes	

4.	NUTRITIONAL PROBLEMS	Complains about the taste of many foods	a.	Leaves 25% or more of food uneaten at most meals	c.
		Regular or repetitive complaints of hunger	b.	NONE OF ABOVE	d.

5.	NUTRITIONAL APPROACHES	(Check all that apply in last 7 days)			
		Parenteral/IV	a.	Dietary supplement between meals	f.
		Feeding tube	b.	Plate guard, stabilized built-up utensil, etc.	g.
		Mechanically altered diet	c.		
		Syringe (oral feeding)	d.	On a planned weight change program	h.
		Therapeutic diet	e.	NONE OF ABOVE	i.

6.	PARENTERAL OR ENTERAL INTAKE	(Skip to Section L if neither 5a nor 5b is checked)
		a. Code the proportion of total calories the resident received through parenteral or tube feedings in the last 7 days
		0. None 3. 51% to 75%
		1. 1% to 25% 4. 76% to 100%
		2. 26% to 50%
		b. Code the average fluid intake per day by IV or tube in last 7 days
		0. None 3. 1001 to 1500 cc/day
		1. 1 to 500 cc/day 4. 1501 to 2000 cc/day
		2. 501 to 1000 cc/day 5. 2001 or more cc/day

SECTION L. ORAL/DENTAL STATUS

1.	ORAL STATUS AND DISEASE PREVENTION	Debris (soft, easily movable substances) present in mouth prior to going to bed at night	a.
		Has dentures or removable bridge	b.
		Some/all natural teeth lost—does not have or does not use dentures (or partial plates)	c.
		Broken, loose, or carious teeth	d.
		Inflamed gums (gingiva); swollen or bleeding gums; oral abcesses; ulcers or rashes	e.
		Daily cleaning of teeth/dentures or daily mouth care—by resident or staff	f.
		NONE OF ABOVE	g.

SECTION M. SKIN CONDITION

1.	ULCERS (Due to any cause)	(Record the number of ulcers at each ulcer stage—regardless of cause. If none present at a stage, record "0" (zero). Code all that apply during last 7 days. Code 9 = 9 or more.) [Requires full body exam.]	Number at Stage
		a. Stage 1. A persistent area of skin redness (without a break in the skin) that does not disappear when pressure is relieved.	
		b. Stage 2. A partial thickness loss of skin layers that presents clinically as an abrasion, blister, or shallow crater.	
		c. Stage 3. A full thickness of skin is lost, exposing the subcutaneous tissues - presents as a deep crater with or without undermining adjacent tissue.	
		d. Stage 4. A full thickness of skin and subcutaneous tissue is lost, exposing muscle or bone.	

2.	TYPE OF ULCER	(For each type of ulcer, code for the highest stage in the last 7 days using scale in item M1—i.e., 0=none; stages 1, 2, 3, 4)	
		a. Pressure ulcer—any lesion caused by pressure resulting in damage of underlying tissue	
		b. Stasis ulcer—open lesion caused by poor circulation in the lower extremities	

3.	HISTORY OF RESOLVED ULCERS	Resident had an ulcer that was resolved or cured in LAST 90 DAYS	
		0. No 1. Yes	

4.	OTHER SKIN PROBLEMS OR LESIONS PRESENT	(Check all that apply during last 7 days)	
		Abrasions, bruises	a.
		Burns (second or third degree)	b.
		Open lesions other than ulcers, rashes, cuts (e.g., cancer lesions)	c.
		Rashes—e.g., intertrigo, eczema, drug rash, heat rash, herpes zoster	d.
		Skin desensitized to pain or pressure	e.
		Skin tears or cuts (other than surgery)	f.
		Surgical wounds	g.
		NONE OF ABOVE	h.

5.	SKIN TREATMENTS	(Check all that apply during last 7 days)	
		Pressure relieving device(s) for chair	a.
		Pressure relieving device(s) for bed	b.
		Turning/repositioning program	c.
		Nutrition or hydration intervention to manage skin problems	d.
		Ulcer care	e.
		Surgical wound care	f.
		Application of dressings (with or without topical medications) other than to feet	g.
		Application of ointments/medications (other than to feet)	h.
		Other preventative or protective skin care (other than to feet)	i.
		NONE OF ABOVE	j.

6.	FOOT PROBLEMS AND CARE	(Check all that apply during last 7 days)	
		Resident has one or more foot problems—e.g., corns, callouses, bunions, hammer toes, overlapping toes, pain, structural problems	a.
		Infection of the foot—e.g., cellulitis, purulent drainage	b.
		Open lesions on the foot	c.
		Nails/calluses trimmed during last 90 days	d.
		Received preventative or protective foot care (e.g., used special shoes, inserts, pads, toe separators)	e.
		Application of dressings (with or without topical medications)	f.
		NONE OF ABOVE	g.

SECTION N. ACTIVITY PURSUIT PATTERNS

1.	TIME AWAKE	(Check appropriate time periods over last 7 days) Resident awake all or most of time (i.e., naps no more than one hour per time period) in the:			
		Morning	a.	Evening	c.
		Afternoon	b.	NONE OF ABOVE	d.

(If resident is comatose, skip to Section O)

2.	AVERAGE TIME INVOLVED IN ACTIVITIES	(When awake and not receiving treatments or ADL care)	
		0. Most—more than 2/3 of time	2. Little—less than 1/3 of time
		1. Some—from 1/3 to 2/3 of time	3. None

3.	PREFERRED ACTIVITY SETTINGS	(Check all settings in which activities are preferred)			
		Own room	a.		
		Day/activity room	b.	Outside facility	d.
		Inside NH/off unit	c.	NONE OF ABOVE	e.

4.	GENERAL ACTIVITY PREFERENCES (adapted to resident's current abilities)	(Check all PREFERENCES whether or not activity is currently available to resident)			
		Cards/other games	a.	Trips/shopping	g.
		Crafts/arts	b.	Walking/wheeling outdoors	h.
		Exercise/sports	c.	Watching TV	i.
		Music	d.	Gardening or plants	j.
		Reading/writing	e.	Talking or conversing	k.
		Spiritual/religious activities	f.	Helping others	l.
				NONE OF ABOVE	m.

MDS 2.0 September, 2000

Resident_____   Numeric Identifier_____

5.	PREFERS CHANGE IN DAILY ROUTINE	Code for resident preferences in daily routines 0. No change 1. Slight change 2. Major change
		a. Type of activities in which resident is currently involved
		b. Extent of resident involvement in activities

SECTION O. MEDICATIONS

1.	NUMBER OF MEDICA-TIONS	(Record the number of different medications used in the last 7 days; enter "0" if none used)	
2.	NEW MEDICA-TIONS	(Resident currently receiving medications that were initiated during the last 90 days) 0. No 1. Yes	
3.	INJECTIONS	(Record the number of DAYS injections of any type received during the last 7 days; enter "0" if none used)	
4.	DAYS RECEIVED THE FOLLOWING MEDICATION	(Record the number of DAYS during last 7 days; enter "0" if not used. Note—enter "1" for long-acting meds used less than weekly)	
		a. Antipsychotic	d. Hypnotic
		b. Antianxiety	e. Diuretic
		c. Antidepressant	

SECTION P. SPECIAL TREATMENTS AND PROCEDURES

1.	SPECIAL TREAT-MENTS, PROCE-DURES, AND PROGRAMS	a. SPECIAL CARE—Check treatments or programs received during the last 14 days			
		TREATMENTS		Ventilator or respirator	l.
		Chemotherapy	a.	**PROGRAMS**	
		Dialysis	b.	Alcohol/drug treatment program	m.
		IV medication	c.	Alzheimer's/dementia special care unit	n.
		Intake/output	d.		
		Monitoring acute medical condition	e.	Hospice care	o.
		Ostomy care	f.	Pediatric unit	p.
		Oxygen therapy	g.	Respite care	q.
		Radiation	h.	Training in skills required to return to the community (e.g., taking medications, house work, shopping, transportation, ADLs)	r.
		Suctioning	i.		
		Tracheostomy care	j.		
		Transfusions	k.	*NONE OF ABOVE*	s.

b. THERAPIES - Record the number of days and total minutes each of the following therapies was administered (for at least 15 minutes a day) in the last 7 calendar days (Enter 0 if none or less than 15 min. daily)
[Note—count only post admission therapies]

(A) = # of days administered for 15 minutes or more (B) = total # of minutes provided in last 7 days	DAYS (A)	MIN (B)
a. Speech - language pathology and audiology services		
b. Occupational therapy		
c. Physical therapy		
d. Respiratory therapy		
e. Psychological therapy (by any licensed mental health professional)		

2.	INTERVEN-TION PROGRAMS FOR MOOD, BEHAVIOR, COGNITIVE LOSS	(Check all interventions or strategies used in last 7 days—no matter where received)	
		Special behavior symptom evaluation program	a.
		Evaluation by a licensed mental health specialist in last 90 days	b.
		Group therapy	c.
		Resident-specific deliberate changes in the environment to address mood/behavior patterns—e.g., providing bureau in which to rummage	d.
		Reorientation—e.g., cueing	e.
		NONE OF ABOVE	f.

3.	NURSING REHABILITA-TION/RESTOR-ATIVE CARE	Record the NUMBER OF DAYS each of the following rehabilitation or restorative techniques or practices was provided to the resident for more than or equal to 15 minutes per day in the last 7 days (Enter 0 if none or less than 15 min. daily.)			
		a. Range of motion (passive)		f. Walking	
		b. Range of motion (active)		g. Dressing or grooming	
		c. Splint or brace assistance		h. Eating or swallowing	
		TRAINING AND SKILL PRACTICE IN:		i. Amputation/prosthesis care	
		d. Bed mobility		j. Communication	
		e. Transfer		k. Other	

4.	DEVICES AND RESTRAINTS	(Use the following codes for last 7 days:) 0. Not used 1. Used less than daily 2. Used daily	
		Bed rails	
		a. — Full bed rails on all open sides of bed	
		b. — Other types of side rails used (e.g., half rail, one side)	
		c. Trunk restraint	
		d. Limb restraint	
		e. Chair prevents rising	
5.	HOSPITAL STAY(S)	Record number of times resident was admitted to hospital with an overnight stay in last 90 days (or since last assessment if less than 90 days). (Enter 0 if no hospital admissions)	
6.	EMERGENCY ROOM (ER) VISIT(S)	Record number of times resident visited ER without an overnight stay in last 90 days (or since last assessment if less than 90 days). (Enter 0 if no ER visits)	
7.	PHYSICIAN VISITS	In the LAST 14 DAYS (or since admission if less than 14 days in facility) how many days has the physician (or authorized assistant or practitioner) examined the resident? (Enter 0 if none)	
8.	PHYSICIAN ORDERS	In the LAST 14 DAYS (or since admission if less than 14 days in facility) how many days has the physician (or authorized assistant or practitioner) changed the resident's orders? Do not include order renewals without change. (Enter 0 if none)	
9.	ABNORMAL LAB VALUES	Has the resident had any abnormal lab values during the last 90 days (or since admission)? 0. No 1. Yes	

SECTION Q. DISCHARGE POTENTIAL AND OVERALL STATUS

1.	DISCHARGE POTENTIAL	a. Resident expresses/indicates preference to return to the community 0. No 1. Yes	
		b. Resident has a support person who is positive towards discharge 0. No 1. Yes	
		c. Stay projected to be of a short duration— discharge projected within 90 days (do not include expected discharge due to death) 0. No 2. Within 31-90 days 1. Within 30 days 3. Discharge status uncertain	
2.	OVERALL CHANGE IN CARE NEEDS	Resident's overall self sufficiency has changed significantly as compared to status of 90 days ago (or since last assessment if less than 90 days) 0. No change 1. Improved—receives fewer supports, needs less restrictive level of care 2. Deteriorated—receives more support	

SECTION R. ASSESSMENT INFORMATION

1.	PARTICIPA-TION IN ASSESS-MENT	a. Resident: 0. No 1. Yes		
		b. Family: 0. No 1. Yes 2. No family		
		c. Significant other: 0. No 1. Yes 2. None		
2.	SIGNATURE OF PERSON COORDINATING THE ASSESSMENT:			

a. Signature of RN Assessment Coordinator (sign on above line)

b. Date RN Assessment Coordinator signed as complete						
	Month		Day		Year	

MDS 2.0 September, 2000

Resident _____   Numeric Identifier _____

SECTION T. THERAPY SUPPLEMENT FOR MEDICARE PPS

1.	**SPECIAL TREAT-MENTS AND PROCE-DURES**	**a. RECREATION THERAPY**—*Enter number of days and total minutes of recreation therapy administered (for at least 15 minutes a day) in the last 7 days (Enter 0 if none)*

	DAYS (A)	MIN (B)
(A) = # of days administered for 15 minutes or more		
(B) = total # of minutes provided in last 7 days		

Skip unless this is a Medicare 5 day or Medicare readmission/return assessment.

b. ORDERED THERAPIES—*Has physician ordered any of following therapies to begin in FIRST 14 days of stay—physical therapy, occupational therapy, or speech pathology service?*
0. No   1. Yes

If not ordered, skip to item 2

c. Through day 15, provide an estimate of the number of days when at least 1 therapy service can be expected to have been delivered.

d. Through day 15, provide an estimate of the number of therapy minutes (across the therapies) that can be expected to be delivered?

2.	**WALKING WHEN MOST SELF SUFFICIENT**	*Complete item 2 if ADL self-performance score for TRANSFER (G.1.b.A) is 0,1,2, or 3 AND at least one of the following are present:*

- Resident received physical therapy involving gait training (P.1.b.c)
- Physical therapy was ordered for the resident involving gait training (T.1.b)
- Resident received nursing rehabilitation for walking (P.3.f)
- Physical therapy involving walking has been discontinued within the past 180 days

Skip to item 3 if resident did not walk in last 7 days

(FOR FOLLOWING FIVE ITEMS, BASE CODING ON THE EPISODE WHEN THE RESIDENT WALKED THE FARTHEST WITHOUT SITTING DOWN. INCLUDE WALKING DURING REHABILITATION SESSIONS.)

a. Furthest distance walked without sitting down during this episode.

0. 150+ feet	3. 10-25 feet
1. 51-149 feet	4. Less than 10 feet
2. 26-50 feet	

b. Time walked without sitting down during this episode.

0. 1-2 minutes	3. 11-15 minutes
1. 3-4 minutes	4. 16-30 minutes
2. 5-10 minutes	5. 31+ minutes

c. Self-Performance in walking during this episode.

0. *INDEPENDENT*—No help or oversight
1. *SUPERVISION*—Oversight, encouragement or cueing provided
2. *LIMITED ASSISTANCE*—Resident highly involved in walking; received physical help in guided maneuvering of limbs or other nonweight bearing assistance
3. *EXTENSIVE ASSISTANCE*—Resident received weight bearing assistance while walking

d. Walking support provided associated with this episode (code regardless of resident's self-performance classification).

0. No setup or physical help from staff
1. Setup help only
2. One person physical assist
3. Two+ persons physical assist

e. Parallel bars used by resident in association with this episode.

0. No   1. Yes

3.	**CASE MIX GROUP**	Medicare		State	

MDS 2.0 September, 2000

SECTION V. RESIDENT ASSESSMENT PROTOCOL SUMMARY   Numeric Identifier _____

Resident's Name:	Medical Record No.:

1. Check if RAP is triggered.

2. For each triggered RAP, use the RAP guidelines to identify areas needing further assessment. Document relevant assessment information regarding the resident's status.

- Describe:
  — Nature of the condition (may include presence or lack of objective data and subjective complaints).
  — Complications and risk factors that affect your decision to proceed to care planning.
  — Factors that must be considered in developing individualized care plan interventions.
  — Need for referrals/further evaluation by appropriate health professionals.

- Documentation should support your decision-making regarding whether to proceed with a care plan for a triggered RAP and the type(s) of care plan interventions that are appropriate for a particular resident.

  - Documentation may appear anywhere in the clinical record (e.g., progress notes, consults, flowsheets, etc.).

3. Indicate under the Location of RAP Assessment Documentation column where information related to the RAP assessment can be found.

4. For each triggered RAP, indicate whether a new care plan, care plan revision, or continuation of current care plan is necessary to address the problem(s) identified in your assessment. The Care Planning Decision column must be completed within 7 days of completing the RAI (MDS and RAPs).

A. RAP PROBLEM AREA	(a) Check if triggered	Location and Date of RAP Assessment Documentation	(b) Care Planning Decision—check if addressed in care plan
1. DELIRIUM			
2. COGNITIVE LOSS			
3. VISUAL FUNCTION			
4. COMMUNICATION			
5. ADL FUNCTIONAL/ REHABILITATION POTENTIAL			
6. URINARY INCONTINENCE AND INDWELLING CATHETER			
7. PSYCHOSOCIAL WELL-BEING			
8. MOOD STATE			
9. BEHAVIORAL SYMPTOMS			
10. ACTIVITIES			
11. FALLS			
12. NUTRITIONAL STATUS			
13. FEEDING TUBES			
14. DEHYDRATION/FLUID MAINTENANCE			
15. DENTAL CARE			
16. PRESSURE ULCERS			
17. PSYCHOTROPIC DRUG USE			
18. PHYSICAL RESTRAINTS			

B.

_____
1. Signature of RN Coordinator for RAP Assessment Process   2. ☐☐ — ☐☐ — ☐☐☐☐
   Month   Day   Year

_____
3. Signature of Person Completing Care Planning Decision   4. ☐☐ — ☐☐ — ☐☐☐☐
   Month   Day   Year

MDS 2.0 September, 2000

MDS QUARTERLY ASSESSMENT FORM

Numeric Identifier _____

A1.	RESIDENT NAME	a. (First) b. (Middle initial) c. (Last) d. (Jr/Sr)
A2.	ROOM NUMBER	☐☐☐☐
A3.	ASSESSMENT REFERENCE DATE	a. Last day of MDS observation period ☐☐ – ☐☐ – ☐☐☐☐ Month – Day – Year b. Original (0) or corrected copy of form (enter number of correction) ☐
A4a	DATE OF REENTRY	Date of reentry from most recent temporary discharge to a hospital in last 90 days (or since last assessment or admission if less than 90 days) ☐☐ – ☐☐ – ☐☐☐☐ Month – Day – Year
A6.	MEDICAL RECORD NO.	☐☐☐☐☐☐☐☐
B1.	COMATOSE	(Persistent vegetative state/no discernible consciousness) 0. No 1. Yes (Skip to Section G) ☐
B2.	MEMORY	(Recall of what was learned or known) a. Short-term memory OK—seems/appears to recall after 5 minutes 0. Memory OK 1. Memory problem ☐ b. Long-term memory OK—seems/appears to recall long past 0. Memory OK 1. Memory problem ☐
B4.	COGNITIVE SKILLS FOR DAILY DECISION-MAKING	(Made decisions regarding tasks of daily life) 0. INDEPENDENT—decisions consistent/reasonable 1. MODIFIED INDEPENDENCE—some difficulty in new situations only 2. MODERATELY IMPAIRED—decisions poor; cues/supervision required 3. SEVERELY IMPAIRED—never/rarely made decisions ☐
B5.	INDICATORS OF DELIRIUM—PERIODIC DISORDERED THINKING/AWARENESS	(Code for behavior in the last 7 days.) [Note: Accurate assessment requires conversations with staff and family who have direct knowledge of resident's behavior over this time]. 0. Behavior not present 1. Behavior present, not of recent onset 2. Behavior present, over last 7 days appears different from resident's usual functioning (e.g., new onset or worsening) a. EASILY DISTRACTED—(e.g., difficulty paying attention; gets sidetracked) ☐ b. PERIODS OF ALTERED PERCEPTION OR AWARENESS OF SURROUNDINGS—(e.g., moves lips or talks to someone not present; believes he/she is somewhere else; confuses night and day) ☐ c. EPISODES OF DISORGANIZED SPEECH—(e.g., speech is incoherent, nonsensical, irrelevant, or rambling from subject to subject; loses train of thought) ☐ d. PERIODS OF RESTLESSNESS—(e.g., fidgeting or picking at skin, clothing, napkins, etc; frequent position changes; repetitive physical movements or calling out) ☐ e. PERIODS OF LETHARGY—(e.g., sluggishness; staring into space; difficult to arouse; little body movement) ☐ f. MENTAL FUNCTION VARIES OVER THE COURSE OF THE DAY—(e.g., sometimes better, sometimes worse; behaviors sometimes present, sometimes not) ☐
C4.	MAKING SELF UNDERSTOOD	(Expressing information content—however able) 0. UNDERSTOOD 1. USUALLY UNDERSTOOD—difficulty finding words or finishing thoughts 2. SOMETIMES UNDERSTOOD—ability is limited to making concrete requests 3. RARELY/NEVER UNDERSTOOD ☐
C6.	ABILITY TO UNDERSTAND OTHERS	(Understanding verbal information content—however able) 0. UNDERSTANDS 1. USUALLY UNDERSTANDS—may miss some part/intent of message 2. SOMETIMES UNDERSTANDS—responds adequately to simple, direct communication 3. RARELY/NEVER UNDERSTANDS ☐
E1.	INDICATORS OF DEPRESSION, ANXIETY, SAD MOOD	(Code for indicators observed in last 30 days, irrespective of the assumed cause) 0. Indicator not exhibited in last 30 days 1. Indicator of this type exhibited up to five days a week 2. Indicator of this type exhibited daily or almost daily (6, 7 days a week) **VERBAL EXPRESSIONS OF DISTRESS** a. Resident made negative statements—e.g., "Nothing matters; Would rather be dead; What's the use; Regrets having lived so long; Let me die" ☐ b. Repetitive questions—e.g., "Where do I go; What do I do?" ☐ c. Repetitive verbalizations—e.g., calling out for help, ("God help me") ☐ d. Persistent anger with self or others—e.g., easily annoyed, anger at placement in nursing home; anger at care received ☐ e. Self deprecation—e.g., "I am nothing; I am of no use to anyone" ☐

E1.	INDICATORS OF DEPRESSION, ANXIETY, SAD MOOD (cont.)	**VERBAL EXPRESSIONS OF DISTRESS** f. Expressions of what appear to be unrealistic fears—e.g., fear of being abandoned, left alone, being with others ☐ g. Recurrent statements that something terrible is about to happen—e.g., believes he or she is about to die, have a heart attack ☐ h. Repetitive health complaints—e.g., persistently seeks medical attention, obsessive concern with body functions ☐ i. Repetitive anxious complaints/concerns (non-health related) e.g., persistently seeks attention/reassurance regarding schedules, meals, laundry, clothing, relationship issues ☐
		SLEEP-CYCLE ISSUES j. Unpleasant mood in morning ☐ k. Insomnia/change in usual sleep pattern ☐ **SAD, APATHETIC, ANXIOUS APPEARANCE** l. Sad, pained, worried facial expressions—e.g., furrowed brows ☐ m. Crying, tearfulness ☐ n. Repetitive physical movements—e.g., pacing, hand wringing, restlessness, fidgeting, picking ☐ **LOSS OF INTEREST** o. Withdrawal from activities of interest—e.g., no interest in long standing activities or being with family/friends ☐ p. Reduced social interaction ☐
E2.	MOOD PERSISTENCE	One or more indicators of depressed, sad or anxious mood were not easily altered by attempts to "cheer up", console, or reassure the resident over last 7 days 0. No mood indicators 1. Indicators present, easily altered 2. Indicators present, not easily altered ☐
E4.	BEHAVIORAL SYMPTOMS	(A) Behavioral symptom frequency in last 7 days 0. Behavior not exhibited in last 7 days 1. Behavior of this type occurred 1 to 3 days in last 7 days 2. Behavior of this type occurred 4 to 6 days, but less than daily 3. Behavior of this type occurred daily (B) Behavioral symptom alterability in last 7 days 0. Behavior not present OR behavior was easily altered 1. Behavior was not easily altered

		(A)	(B)
a.	WANDERING (moved with no rational purpose, seemingly oblivious to needs or safety)	☐	☐
b.	VERBALLY ABUSIVE BEHAVIORAL SYMPTOMS (others were threatened, screamed at, cursed at)	☐	☐
c.	PHYSICALLY ABUSIVE BEHAVIORAL SYMPTOMS (others were hit, shoved, scratched, sexually abused)	☐	☐
d.	SOCIALLY INAPPROPRIATE/DISRUPTIVE BEHAVIORAL SYMPTOMS (made disruptive sounds, noisiness, screaming, self-abusive acts, sexual behavior or disrobing in public, smeared/threw food/feces, hoarding, rummaged through others' belongings)	☐	☐
e.	RESISTS CARE (resisted taking medications/injections, ADL assistance, or eating)	☐	☐

G1.	(A) ADL SELF-PERFORMANCE—(Code for resident's PERFORMANCE OVER ALL SHIFTS during last 7 days—Not including setup)
	0. INDEPENDENT—No help or oversight —OR— Help/oversight provided only 1 or 2 times during last 7 days 1. SUPERVISION—Oversight, encouragement or cueing provided 3 or more times during last 7 days —OR— Supervision (3 or more times) plus physical assistance provided only 1 or 2 times during last 7 days 2. LIMITED ASSISTANCE—Resident highly involved in activity; received physical help in guided maneuvering of limbs or other nonweight bearing assistance 3 or more times—OR—More help provided only 1 or 2 times during last 7 days 3. EXTENSIVE ASSISTANCE—While resident performed part of activity, over last 7-day period, help of following type(s) provided 3 or more times: —Weight-bearing support —Full staff performance during part (but not all) of last 7 days 4. TOTAL DEPENDENCE—Full staff performance of activity during entire 7 days 8. ACTIVITY DID NOT OCCUR during entire 7 days

			(A)
a.	BED MOBILITY	How resident moves to and from lying position, turns side to side, and positions body while in bed	☐
b.	TRANSFER	How resident moves between surfaces—to/from: bed, chair, wheelchair, standing position (EXCLUDE to/from bath/toilet)	☐
c.	WALK IN ROOM	How resident walks between locations in his/her room.	☐
d.	WALK IN CORRIDOR	How resident walks in corridor on unit.	☐
e.	LOCOMOTION ON UNIT	How resident moves between locations in his/her room and adjacent corridor on same floor. If in wheelchair, self-sufficiency once in chair	☐
f.	LOCOMOTION OFF UNIT	How resident moves to and returns from off unit locations (e.g., areas set aside for dining, activities, or treatments). If facility has only one floor, how resident moves to and from distant areas on the floor. If in wheelchair, self-sufficiency once in chair	☐
g.	DRESSING	How resident puts on, fastens, and takes off all items of street clothing, including donning/removing prosthesis	☐
h.	EATING	How resident eats and drinks (regardless of skill). Includes intake of nourishment by other means (e.g., tube feeding, total parenteral nutrition).	☐

MDS 2.0 September, 2000

Resident_____   Numeric Identifier_____

I.	TOILET USE	How resident uses the toilet room (or commode, bedpan, urinal); transfer on/off toilet, cleanses, changes pad, manages ostomy or catheter, adjusts clothes
J.	PERSONAL HYGIENE	How resident maintains personal hygiene, including combing hair, brushing teeth, shaving, applying makeup, washing/drying face, hands, and perineum (EXCLUDE baths and showers)

G2. BATHING — How resident takes full-body bath/shower, sponge bath, and transfers in/out of tub/shower (EXCLUDE washing of back and hair.) *Code for most dependent in self-performance.* (A) BATHING SELF PERFORMANCE codes appear below

0. Independent—No help provided
1. Supervision—Oversight help only
2. Physical help limited to transfer only
3. Physical help in part of bathing activity
4. Total dependence
8. Activity itself did not occur during entire 7 days

(A)

G4. FUNCTIONAL LIMITATION IN RANGE OF MOTION (Code for limitations during last 7 days that interfered with daily functions or placed residents at risk of injury)

(A) RANGE OF MOTION
0. No limitation
1. Limitation on one side
2. Limitation on both sides

(B) VOLUNTARY MOVEMENT
0. No loss
1. Partial loss
2. Full loss

(A) (B)

a. Neck
b. Arm—Including shoulder or elbow
c. Hand—Including wrist or fingers
d. Leg—Including hip or knee
e. Foot—Including ankle or toes
f. Other limitation or loss

G6. MODES OF TRANSFER (Check all that apply during last 7 days)
a. Bedfast all or most of time   NONE OF ABOVE f.
b. Bed rails used for bed mobility or transfer

H1. CONTINENCE SELF-CONTROL CATEGORIES (Code for resident's PERFORMANCE OVER ALL SHIFTS)
0. CONTINENT—Complete control [includes use of indwelling urinary catheter or ostomy device that does not leak urine or stool]
1. USUALLY CONTINENT—BLADDER, incontinent episodes once a week or less; BOWEL, less than weekly
2. OCCASIONALLY INCONTINENT—BLADDER, 2 or more times a week but not daily; BOWEL, once a week
3. FREQUENTLY INCONTINENT—BLADDER, tended to be incontinent daily, but some control present (e.g., on day shift); BOWEL, 2-3 times a week
4. INCONTINENT—Had inadequate control BLADDER, multiple daily episodes; BOWEL, all (or almost all) of the time

a. BOWEL CONTINENCE — Control of bowel movement, with appliance or bowel continence programs, if employed
b. BLADDER CONTINENCE — Control of urinary bladder function (if dribbles, volume insufficient to soak through underpants), with appliances (e.g., foley) or continence programs, if employed

H2. BOWEL ELIMINATION PATTERN — Fecal impaction d.   NONE OF ABOVE e.

H3. APPLIANCES AND PROGRAMS
a. Any scheduled toileting plan   d. Indwelling catheter
b. Bladder retraining program   i. Ostomy present
c. External (condom) catheter   j. NONE OF ABOVE

I2. INFECTIONS — Urinary tract infection in last 30 days j.   NONE OF ABOVE m.

I3. OTHER CURRENT DIAGNOSES AND ICD-9 CODES (Include only those diseases diagnosed in the last 90 days that have a relationship to current ADL status, cognitive status, mood or behavior status, medical treatments, nursing monitoring, or risk of death)
a. _____ | | | . | |
b. _____ | | | . | |

J1. PROBLEM CONDITIONS (Check all problems present in last 7 days)
Dehydrated; output exceeds input c.   Hallucinations i.
NONE OF ABOVE p.

J2. PAIN SYMPTOMS (Code the highest level of pain present in the last 7 days)
a. FREQUENCY with which resident complains or shows evidence of pain
0. No pain (skip to J4)
1. Pain less than daily
2. Pain daily

b. INTENSITY of pain
1. Mild pain
2. Moderate pain
3. Times when pain is horrible or excrutiating

J4. ACCIDENTS (Check all that apply)
Fell in past 30 days a.   Hip fracture in last 180 days c.
Fell in past 31-180 days b.   Other fracture in last 180 days d.
NONE OF ABOVE e.

J5. STABILITY OF CONDITIONS
a. Conditions/diseases make resident's cognitive, ADL, mood or behavior status unstable—(fluctuating, precarious, or deteriorating)
b. Resident experiencing an acute episode or a flare-up of a recurrent or chronic problem
c. End-stage disease, 6 or fewer months to live
d. NONE OF ABOVE

K3. WEIGHT CHANGE
a. Weight loss—5 % or more in last 30 days; or 10 % or more in last 180 days   0. No   1. Yes
b. Weight gain—5 % or more in last 30 days; or 10 % or more in last 180 days   0. No   1. Yes

K5. NUTRITIONAL APPROACHES
b. Feeding tube
h. On a planned weight change program
L. NONE OF ABOVE

M1. ULCERS (Due to any cause) (Record the number of ulcers at each ulcer stage—regardless of cause. If none present at a stage, record "0" (zero). Code all that apply during last 7 days. Code 9 = 9 or more.) [Requires full body exam.] Number at Stage
a. Stage 1. A persistent area of skin redness (without a break in the skin) that does not disappear when pressure is relieved.
b. Stage 2. A partial thickness loss of skin layers that presents clinically as an abrasion, blister, or shallow crater.
c. Stage 3. A full thickness of skin is lost, exposing the subcutaneous tissues - presents as a deep crater with or without undermining adjacent tissue.
d. Stage 4. A full thickness of skin and subcutaneous tissue is lost, exposing muscle or bone.

M2. TYPE OF ULCER (For each type of ulcer, code for the highest stage in the last 7 days using scale in item M1—i.e., 0=none; stages 1, 2, 3, 4)
a. Pressure ulcer—any lesion caused by pressure resulting in damage of underlying tissue
b. Stasis ulcer—open lesion caused by poor circulation in the lower extremities

N1. TIME AWAKE (Check appropriate time periods over last 7 days) Resident awake all or most of time (i.e., naps no more than one hour per time period) in the:
Morning a.   Evening c.
Afternoon b.   NONE OF ABOVE d.

(If resident is comatose, skip to Section O)

N2. AVERAGE TIME INVOLVED IN ACTIVITIES (When awake and not receiving treatments or ADL care)
0. Most—more than 2/3 of time   2. Little—less than 1/3 of time
1. Some—from 1/3 to 2/3 of time   3. None

O1. NUMBER OF MEDICATIONS (Record the number of different medications used in the last 7 days; enter "0" if none used)

O4. DAYS RECEIVED THE FOLLOWING MEDICATION (Record the number of DAYS during last 7 days; enter "0" if not used. Note—enter "1" for long-acting meds used less than weekly)
a. Antipsychotic   d. Hypnotic
b. Antianxiety   e. Diuretic
c. Antidepressant

P4. DEVICES AND RESTRAINTS Use the following codes for last 7 days:
0. Not used
1. Used less than daily
2. Used daily
Bed rails
a. — Full bed rails on all open sides of bed
b. — Other types of side rails used (e.g., half rail, one side)
c. Trunk restraint
d. Limb restraint
e. Chair prevents rising

Q2. OVERALL CHANGE IN CARE NEEDS Resident's overall level of self sufficiency has changed significantly as compared to status of 90 days ago (or since last assessment if less than 90 days)
0. No change   1. Improved—receives fewer supports, needs less restrictive level of care   2. Deteriorated—receives more support

R2. SIGNATURE OF PERSON COORDINATING THE ASSESSMENT:
a. Signature of RN Assessment Coordinator (sign on above line)
b. Date RN Assessment Coordinator signed as complete   [ ][ ]—[ ][ ]—[ ][ ][ ][ ]   Month Day Year

MDS 2.0 September, 2000

RESIDENT ASSESSMENT PROTOCOL: ACTIVITIES

I.   PROBLEM

The Activities RAP targets residents for whom a revised activity care plan may be required to identify those residents whose inactivity may be a major complication in their lives. Resident capabilities may not be fully recognized: the resident may have recently moved into the facility or staff may have focused too heavily on the instrumental needs of the resident and may have lost sight of complications in the institutional environment.

Resident involvement in passive as well as active activities can be as important in the nursing home as it was in the community. The capabilities of the average resident have obviously been altered as abilities and expectations change, disease intervenes, situational opportunities become less frequent, and extended social relationships less common. But something that should never be overlooked is the great variability within the resident population: many will have ADL deficits, but few will be totally dependent; impaired cognition will be widespread, but so will the ability to apply old skills and learn new ones; and sense may be impaired, but some type of two-way communication is almost always possible.

For the nursing home, activity planning is a universal need. For this RAP, the focus is on cases where the system may have failed the resident, or where the resident has distressing conditions that warrant review of the activity care plan. The types of cases that will be triggered are: (1) residents who have indicated a desire for additional activity choices; (2) cognitively intact, distressed residents who may benefit from an enriched activity program; (3) cognitively deficient, distressed residents whose activity levels should be evaluated; and (4) highly involved residents whose health may be in jeopardy because of their failure to slow down.

In evaluating triggered cases, the following general questions may be helpful:

- *Is inactivity disproportionate to the resident's physical/cognitive abilities or limitations?*
- *Have decreased demands of nursing home life removed the need to make decisions, to set schedules, to meet challenges? Have these changes contributed to resident apathy?*
- *What is the nature of the naturally occurring physical and mental challenges the resident experiences in everyday life?*
- *In what activities is the resident involved? Is he/she normally an active participant in the life of the unit? Is the resident reserved, but actively aware of what is going on around him/her? Or is he/she unaware of sur-*

roundings and activities that take place?
- *Are there proven ways to extend the resident's inquisitive/active engagement in activities?*
- *Might simple staff actions expedite resident involvement in activities? For example: Can equipment be modified to permit greater resident access of the unit? Can the resident's location or position be changed to permit greater access to people, views, or programs? Can time and/or distance limitations for activities be made less demanding without destroying the challenge? Can staff modes of interacting with the resident be more accommodating, possibly less threatening, to resident deficits?*

II. TRIGGERS

ACTIVITIES TRIGGER A (Revise)

Consider revising activity plan if one or more of following present:

> Involved in activities little or none of time
>> [N2 = 2, 3]
> Prefers change in daily routine
>> [N5a = 1, 2][N5b = 1, 2]

ACTIVITIES TRIGGERS B (Review)

Review of activity plan suggested if both of following present:

> Awake all or most of time in morning
>> [N1a = checked]
> Involved in activities most of time
>> N2 = 0]

III. GUIDELINES

The follow up review looks for factors that may impede resident involvement in activities. Although many factors can play a role, age as a valid impediment to participation can normally be ruled out. If age continues to be linked as a major cause of lack of participation, a staff education program may prove effective in remedying what may be overprotective staff behavior.

Issues to be Considered as Activity Plan is Developed.

Is Resident Suitable Challenged, Overstimulated? To some extent, competence depends on environmental demands. When the challenge is not sufficiently demanding, a resident can become bored, perhaps withdrawn, may resort to fault-finding and perhaps even behave mischievously to relieve the boredom.

Eventually, such a resident may become less competent because of the lack of challenge. In contrast, when the resident lacks the competence to meet challenges presented by the surroundings, he or she may react with anger and aggressiveness.

- *Do available activities correspond to resident lifetime values, attitudes, and expectations?*
- *Does resident consider leisure activities a waste of time - he/she never really learned to play, or to do things just for enjoyment?*
- *Have the resident's wishes and prior activity patterns been considered by activity and nursing professionals?*
- *Have staff considered how activities requiring lower energy levels may be of interest to the resident - e.g., reading a book, talking with family and friends, watching the world go by, knitting?*
- *Does the resident have cognitive/functional deficits that either reduce options or preclude involvement in all/most activities that would otherwise have been of interest to him/her?*

Confounding Problems to be Considered.

Health-related factors that may affect participation in activities. Diminished cardiac output, an acute illness, reduced energy reserves, and impaired respiratory function are some of the many reasons that activity level may decline. Most of these conditions need not necessarily incapacitate the resident. All too often, disease-induced reduction of activity may lead to progressive decline through disuse, and further decrease in activity levels. However, this pattern can be broken: many activities can be continued if they are adapted to require less exertion or if the resident is helped in adapting to a lost limb, decreased communication skills, new appliances, and so forth.

- *Is the resident suffering from an acute health problem?*
- *Is resident hindered because of embarrassment/unease due to presence of health-related equipment (tubes, oxygen tank, colostomy bag, wheelchair)?*
- *Has the resident recovered from an illness? Is the capacity for participation in activities greater?*
- *Has an illness left the resident with some disability (e.g., slurred speech, necessity for use of cane/walker/wheelchair, limited use of hands)?*
- *Does resident's treatment regimen allow little time or energy for participation in preferred activities?*

Other Issues to be Considered

Recent decline, in resident status - cognition, communication, function, mood, or behavior. When pathologic changes occur in any aspect of the resident's competence, the pleasurable challenge of activities may narrow. Of special interest are problematic changes that may be related to the use of psychoactive medications.

When residents or staff overreact to such losses, compensatory strategies may be helpful - e.g., impaired residents may benefit from periods of both activity and rest; task segmentation can be considered; or available resident energies can be reserved for pleasurable activities (e.g., using usual stamina reserves to walk to the card room, rather than the bathroom) or activities that have individual significance (e.g., sitting unattended at a daily prayer service rather than at group activity program).

- *Has staff or the resident been overprotective? Or have they misread the seriousness of resident cognitive/functional decline? In what ways?*
- *Has the resident retained skills, or the capacity to learn new skills, sufficient to permit greater activity involvement?*
- *Does staff know what the resident was like prior to the most recent decline? has the physical/other staff offered a prognosis for the resident's future recovery, or change of continued decline?*
- *Is there any substantial reason to believe that the resident cannot tolerate or would be harmed by increased activity levels? What reasons support a counter opinion?*
- *Does resident retain any desire to learn or master a specific new activity? Is this realistic?*
- *Has there been a lack of participation in the majority of activities which he/she stated as preference are as even though these types of activities are provided?*

Environmental factors. Environmental factors include recent changes in resident location, facility rules, season of the year, and physical space limitations that hinder effective resident involvement.

- *Does the interplay of personal, social, and physical aspects of the facility's environment hamper involvement in activities? How might this be addressed?*
- *Are current activity levels affected by the season of the year or the nature of the weather during the MDS assessment period?*
- *Can the resident choose to participate in or to create an activity? How is this influenced by facility rules?*
- *Does resident prefer to be with others, but the physical layout of the unit gets in the way? Do other features in the physical plant frustrate the resident's desire to be involved in the life of the facility? What corrective actions are possible? Have any been taken?*

Changes in availability of family/friends/staff support. Many residents will experience not only a change in resident but also a loss of relationships. When this occurs, staff may wish to consider ways for resident to develop a supportive relationship with another resident, staff member or volunteer that may increase the desire to socialize with others and/or to participate in activities with this new friend.

- *Has a staff person who has been instrumental in involving a resident in activities left the facility/been reassigned?*
- *Is a new member in a group activity viewed by a resident as taking over?*
- *Has another resident who was a leader on the unit died or left the unit?*
- *Is resident shy, unable to make new friends?*
- *Does resident's expression of dissatisfaction with fellow residents indicate he/she does not want to be a part of an activities group?*

Possible Confounding Problems to be considered for Those Now Actively Involved in Activities. Of special interest are cardiac and other diseases that might suggest a need to slow down.

ACTIVITIES RAP KEY (For MDS Version 2.0)

TRIGGERS - REVISION	GUIDELINES
ACTIVITIES TRIGGER A (Revise) Consider revising activity plan if one or more of the following present: • Involved in activities little or none of time [N2 = 2,3] • Prefers change in daily routine [N5a = 1,2] [N5b = 1,2] **ACTIVITIES TRIGGERS B (Review)** Review of activity plan suggested if both of following present • Awake all or most of time in morning [N1 = a] • Involved in activities most of time [N2 = 0]	Issues to be considered as activity plan is developed: • Time in facility [AB1] • Cognitive status [B2, B4] • Walking/locomotion pattern [G1c,d,e,f] • Unstable/acute health conditions [J5a,b] • Number of treatments received [P1] • Use of Psychoactive medications [O4a,b,c,d] Confounding problems to be considered: • Performs tasks slowly and at different levels (reduced energy reserves) [G8c,d] • Cardiac dysrhythmias [I1e] • Hypertension [I1h] • CVA [I1t] • Respiratory diseases [I1hh, I1ii] • Pain [J2] Other issues to be considered • Customary routines [AC] • Mood [E1. E2] and Behavioral Symptoms [E4] • Recent loss of close family member/friend or staff [F2f; from record] • Whether daily routine is very different from prior pattern in the community [F3c]

REFERENCES TO FEDERAL REGULATIONS

RESOURCES

State Operations Manual (Pub 100-7) Appendix PP Centers for Medicare and Medicaid, Revision 5, 6-1-2006 http://www.hhs.gov/manuals.

Long Term Care Facility Resident Assessment Instrument (RAI) User's Manual, MDS. 2.0, Centers for Medicare and Medicaid, Update March, 2007 http//www.cms.hhs.gov/medicaid/mds20.

Nursing Home Compare (Website for consumer information and quality measures for facilities) Centers for Medicare and Medicaid, http//www.medicare.gov/NHCompare.

Summary of Key Points for Documentation of Activity Programs

F249 Qualifications of Activity Professional

A. Intent:
1. The activity program is directed by a qualified professional.

B. Definition:
   1. "Recognized accrediting body" refers to those organizations that certify, register, or license therapeutic recreation specialists, activity professionals, or occupational therapists.

C. Activities Director Responsibilities
   1. Directs the development, implementation, supervision and ongoing evaluation of the activity program.
   2. Completes the activities component of the comprehensive assessment.
   3. Contributing to the comprehensive care plan, goals and approaches that are individualized to match the skills, abilities, and interest/preferences of each resident.
   4. Scheduling of activities, both individual and groups
   5. Implementing or delegating implementation of the programs.
   6. Monitoring the response and reviewing/evaluating the response to the programs to determine if the activities meet the assessed needs of the resident
   7. Making revisions to the activity program and to individual resident care plans as necessary.

D. Criteria for Compliance.
   The facility is in compliance with this requirement if they:
   1. Have employed a qualifies professional to provide direction in the development and implementation of activities in accordance with resident needs and goals, and the director:
   a. Has completed or delegated the completion of the activities component of the comprehensive assessment
   b. Contributed or directed the contribution to the comprehensive care plan of activity goals and approaches that are individualized to match the skills, abilities, and interests/preferences of each resident
   c. Has monitored and evaluated the resident's response to activities and revised the approaches as appropriate; and
   d. Has developed, implemented, supervised and evaluated the activities program.

F248 Activities

A. Intent:
1. The facility identifies each resident's interest and needs; and
2. The facility involves the resident in an ongoing program of activities that is designed to appeal to his or her interests and to enhance the resident's highest practicable level of physical, mental and psychosocial well-being.

B. Definitions:
1. "Activities" any endeavor, other than routine ADLs, in which a resident participates that is intended to enhance her/his sense of well-being and to promote or enhance physical, cognitive and emotional health. These include, but are not limited to, activities that promote self-esteem, pleasure, comfort, education creativity, success, and independence.
2. "One to One Programming" provided to residents who will not, or cannot, effectively plan their own activity pursuits, or residents needing specialized or extended programs to enhance their overall daily routine and activity pursuit needs.
3. "Person Appropriate" refers to the idea that each resident has a person identity and history that involves more than just their medical illnesses or functional impairments. Activities should be relevant to the specific needs, interests, culture, background, etc. of the individual for whom they are developed.
4. "Program of Activities" a combination of large and small group, one-to-one, and self-directed activities; and a system that supports the development, implementation, and evaluation of the activities provided to the residents in the facility.

C. Assessment:
1. Activity pursuit patterns, preferences, longstanding interests and customary routines
2. How the resident's current physical, mental and psychosocial health status affects her/his choice of activities and her/his ability to participate.
a. Skills, abilities, strengths, personal goals
b. Accommodation of needs to allow participation
3. Specific information how the resident prefers to participate in activities
4. Current needs for special adaptations in order to participate in desired activities
5. Need for time-limited participation, such as short attention span or illness that permits only limited time out of bed.
6. Resident's desired daily routine and availability of activities; and
7. Resident's choices for group, one-to-one and self-directed activities.
8. Any significant changes in activity patterns before or after admission.
9. NOTE: Some resident may be independently capable of pursuing their own activities without intervention from the facility. This information should be noted in the assessment and identified in the care plan.

D.   Care Planning:
      1.   Problem/Need Statements:
      a.   Person appropriate
      b.   Resident's interests, preferences, abilities
      c.   Issues affecting the resident's involvement/engagement in activities,
2.   Goals:
      a.   Measurable objectives
      b.   Desired Outcomes
3.   Interventions with identification of responsible disciplines (examples)
      a.   Notifying residents of preferred activities
      b.   Transporting residents who need assistance to and from activities (including indoor, outdoor and outings)
      c.   Providing needed functional assistance (toileting and eating assistance)
      d.   Supplies and adaptations such as obtaining and returning audio books, setting up adaptive equipment.
      e.   Timing of administration of medications (such as diuretics) to avoid interfering with resident's ability to participate.
      f.   Timing of administration of pain medication to allow the medication to take effect prior to an activity the resident enjoys.
      g.   Continuation of life roles, consistent with resident preferences and functional capacity (continue work or hobbies)
      h.   Development of new interests, hobbies and skills
      i.   Connecting with the community, worship, support groups, athletic and educational, outings.
      j.   Altering therapy or bath/shower schedule to make it possible to attend an activity
      k.   Assisting resident to get to and participate in desired activity (dressing, toileting, transportation)
      l.   Providing supplies and assistance during weekends, nights, holidays, evenings, or when the activities staff are unavailable.
      m.   Providing late breakfast to allow a resident to continue a lifelong pattern of attending religious services before eating.
      n.   Many activities can be adapted in various ways to accommodate the resident's change in functioning due to physical or cognitive limitations.

E.   Criteria for Compliance
      The facility is in compliance with this requirement if they:
      1.   Recognized and assessed for preferences, choices, specific conditions, causes and/or problems, needs and behaviors.
      2.   Defined and implemented activities in accordance with resident needs and goals;
      3.   Monitored and evaluated the resident's response; and
      4.   Revised the approaches as appropriate.

Surveyor Guidelines State Operations Manual 100-7 Appendix PP

F248 §483.15(f) Activities **Revised 6/1/2006**

§483.15(f)(1) The facility must provide for an ongoing program of activities designed to meet, in accordance with the comprehensive assessment, the interests and the physical, mental, and psychosocial well?being of each resident.

INTENT: §483.15(f)(1) Activities

The intent of this requirement is that:

- The facility identifies each resident's interests and needs; and

- The facility involves the resident in an ongoing program of activities that is designed to appeal to his or her interests and to enhance the resident's highest practicable level of physical, mental, and psychosocial well-being.

DEFINITIONS

Definitions are provided to clarify key terms used in this guidance.

- "Activities" refer to any endeavor, other than routine ADLs, in which a resident participates that is intended to enhance her/his sense of well-being and to promote or enhance physical, cognitive, and emotional health. These include, but are not limited to, activities that promote self-esteem, pleasure, comfort, education, creativity, success, and independence.

    NOTE: ADL-related activities, such as manicures/pedicures, hair styling, and makeovers, may be considered part of the activities program.

- "One-to-One Programming" refers to programming provided to residents who will not, or cannot, effectively plan their own activity pursuits, or residents needing specialized or extended programs to enhance their overall daily routine and activity pursuit needs.

- "Person Appropriate" refers to the idea that each resident has a personal identity and history that involves more than just their medical illnesses or functional impairments. Activities should be relevant to the specific needs, interests, culture, background, etc. of the individual for whom they are developed.

- "Program of Activities" includes a combination of large and small group, one-to-one, and self-directed activities; and a system that supports the development, implementation, and evaluation of the activities provided to the residents in the facility.[1]

OVERVIEW

In long term care, an ongoing program of activities refers to the provision of activities in accordance with and based upon an individual resident's comprehensive assessment. The Institute of Medicine (IOM)'s 1986 report, "Improving the Quality of Care in Nursing Homes," became the basis for the "Nursing Home Reform" part of OBRA '87 and the current OBRA long term care regulations. The IOM Report identified the need for residents in nursing homes to receive care and/or services to maximize their highest practicable quality of life. However, defining "quality of life" has been difficult, as it is subjective for each person. Thus, it is important for the facility to conduct an individualized assessment of each resident to provide additional opportunities to help enhance a resident's self-esteem and dignity.

Research findings and the observations of positive resident outcomes confirm that activities are an integral component of residents' lives. Residents have indicated that daily life and involvement should be meaningful. Activities are meaningful when they reflect a person's interests and lifestyle, are enjoyable to the person, help the person to feel useful, and provide a sense of belonging.[2]

Residents' Views on Activities

Activities are relevant and valuable to residents' quality of life. In a large-scale study commissioned by CMS, 160 residents in 40 nursing homes were interviewed about what quality of life meant to them. The study found that residents "overwhelmingly assigned priority to dignity, although they labeled this concern in many ways." The researchers determined that the two main components of dignity, in the words of these residents, were "independence" and "positive self-image." Residents listed, under the categories of independence and positive self-image, the elements of "choice of activities" and "activities that amount to something," such as those that produce or teach something; activities using skills from residents' former work; religious activities; and activities that contribute to the nursing home.

The report stated that, "Residents not only discussed particular activities that gave them a sense of purpose but also indicated that a lack of appropriate activities contributes to having no sense of purpose." "Residents rarely mentioned participating in activities as a way to just 'keep busy' or just to socialize. . .The relevance of the activities to the residents' lives must be considered."

According to the study, residents wanted a variety of activities, including those that are not childish, require thinking (such as word games), are gender-specific, produce something useful, relate to previous work of residents, allow for socializing with visitors and participating in community events, and are physically active. The study found that the above concepts were relevant to both interviewable and non-interviewable residents. Researchers observed that non-interviewable residents appeared "happier" and "less agitated" in homes with many planned activities for them.

Non-traditional Approaches to Activities

Surveyors need to be aware that some facilities may take a non-traditional approach to activities. In neighborhoods/households, all staff may be trained as nurse aides and are responsible to provide activities, and activities may resemble those of a private home.[3] Residents, staff, and families may interact in ways that reflect daily life, instead of in formal activities programs. Residents may be more involved in the ongoing activities in their living area, such as care-planned approaches including chores, preparing foods, meeting with other residents to choose spontaneous activities, and leading an activity. It has been reported that, "some culture changed homes might not have a traditional activities calendar, and instead focus on community life to include activities. Instead of an "activities director," some homes have a Community Life Coordinator, a Community Developer, or other title for the individual directing the activities program.[4]

For more information on activities in homes changing to a resident-directed culture, the following websites are available as resources: www.pioneernetwork.net; www.culturechangenow.com; www.qualitypartnersri.org (click on nursing homes); and www.edenalt.com.

ASSESSMENT

The information gathered through the assessment process should be used to develop the activities component of the comprehensive care plan. The ongoing program of activities should match the skills, abilities, needs, and preferences of each resident with the demands of the activity and the characteristics of the physical, social and cultural environments.[5]

In order to develop individualized care planning goals and approaches, the facility should obtain sufficient, detailed information (even if the Activities RAP is not triggered) to determine what activities the resident prefers and what adaptations, if any, are needed.[6] The facility may use, but need not duplicate, information from other sources, such as the RAI, including the RAPs, assessments by other disciplines, observation, and resident and family interviews. Other sources of relevant information include the resident's lifelong interests, spirituality, life roles, goals, strengths, needs and activity pursuit patterns and preferences.[7] This assessment should be completed by or under the supervision of a qualified professional (see F249 for definition of qualified professional).

> NOTE: Some residents may be independently capable of pursuing their own activities without intervention from the facility. This information should be noted in the assessment and identified in the plan of care.

CARE PLANNING

Care planning involves identification of the resident's interests, preferences, and abilities; and any issues, concerns, problems, or needs affecting the resident's involvement/ engagement in activities.[8]   In addition to the activities component of the comprehensive care plan, information may also be found in a separate activity plan, on a CNA flow sheet, in a progress note, etc.

Activity goals related to the comprehensive care plan should be based on measurable objectives and focused on desired outcomes (e.g., engagement in an activity that matches the resident's ability, maintaining attention to the activity for a specified period of time, expressing satisfaction with the activity verbally or non-verbally), not merely on attendance at a certain number of activities per week.

> NOTE: For residents with no discernable response, service provision is still expected and may include one-to-one activities such as talking to the resident, reading to the resident about prior interests, or applying lotion while stroking the resident's hands or feet.

Activities can occur at any time, are not limited to formal activities being provided only by activities staff, and can include activities provided by other facility staff, volunteers, visitors, residents, and family members. All relevant departments should collaborate to develop and implement an individualized activities program for each resident.

Some medications, such as diuretics, or conditions such as pain, incontinence, etc. may affect the resident's participation in activities. Therefore, additional steps may be needed to facilitate the resident's participation in activities, such as:

- If not contraindicated, timing the administration of medications, to the extent possible, to avoid interfering with the resident's ability to participate or to remain at a scheduled activity; or

- If not contraindicated, modifying the administration time of pain medication to allow the medication to take effect prior to an activity the resident enjoys.

The care plan should also identify the discipline(s) that will carry out the approaches. For example:

- Notifying residents of preferred activities;

- Transporting residents who need assistance to and from activities (including indoor, outdoor, and outings);

- Providing needed functional assistance (such as toileting and eating assistance); and

- Providing needed supplies or adaptations, such as obtaining and returning audio books, setting up adaptive equipment, etc.

Concepts the facility should have considered in the development of the activities component of the resident's comprehensive care plan include the following, as applicable to the resident:

- A continuation of life roles, consistent with resident preferences and functional capacity (e.g., to continue work or hobbies such as cooking, table setting, repairing small appliances)[9];

- Encouraging and supporting the development of new interests, hobbies, and skills (e.g., training on using the Internet); and

- Connecting with the community, such as places of worship, veterans' groups, volunteer groups, support groups, wellness groups, athletic or educational connections (via outings or invitations to outside groups to visit the facility).

The facility may need to consider accommodations in schedules, supplies and timing in order to optimize a resident's ability to participate in an activity of choice. Examples of accommodations may include, but are not limited to:

- Altering a therapy or a bath/shower schedule to make it possible for a resident to attend a desired activity that occurs at the same time as the therapy session or bath;

- Assisting residents, as needed, to get to and participate in desired activities (e.g., dressing, toileting, transportation);

- Providing supplies (e.g., books/magazines, music, craft projects, cards, sorting materials) for activities, and assistance when needed, for residents' use (e.g., during weekends, nights, holidays, evenings, or when the activities staff are unavailable); and

- Providing a late breakfast to allow a resident to continue a lifelong pattern of attending religious services before eating.

INTERVENTIONS

The concept of individualized intervention has evolved over the years. Many activity professionals have abandoned generic interventions such as "reality orientation" and large-group activities that include residents with different levels of strengths and needs. In their place, individualized interventions have been developed based upon the assessment of the resident's history, preferences, strengths, and needs. These interventions have changed from the idea of "age-appropriate" activities to promoting "person-appropriate" activities. For example, one person may care for a doll or stroke a stuffed animal, another person may be inclined to reminisce about dolls or stuffed animals they once had, while someone else may enjoy petting a dog but will not be interested in inanimate objects. The surveyor observing these interventions should determine if the facility selected them in response to the resident's history and preferences. Many activities can be adapted in various ways to accommodate the resident's change in functioning due to physical or cognitive limitations.

Some Possible Adaptations that May be Made by the Facility [10, 11]

When evaluating the provision of activities, it is important for the surveyor to identify whether the resident has conditions and/or issues for which staff should have provided adaptations. Examples of adaptations for specific conditions include, but are not limited to the following:

- For the resident with visual impairments: higher levels of lighting without glare; magnifying glasses, light-filtering lenses, telescopic glasses; use of "clock method" to describe where items are located; description of sizes, shapes, colors; large print items including playing cards, newsprint, books; audio books;

- For the resident with hearing impairments: small group activities; placement of resident near speaker/activity leader; use of amplifiers or headphones; decreased background noise; written instructions; use of gestures or sign language to enhance verbal communication; adapted TV (closed captioning, magnified screen, earphones);

- For the resident who has physical limitations, the use of adaptive equipment, proper seating and positioning, placement of supplies and materials[12] (based on clinical assessment and referral as appropriate) to enhance:

  o   Visual interaction and to compensate for loss of visual field (hemianopsia);

  o   Upper extremity function and range of motion (reach);

  o   Hand dexterity (e.g., adapted size of items such as larger handles for cooking and woodworking equipment, built-up paintbrush handles, large needles for crocheting);

  o   The ability to manipulate an item based upon the item's weight, such as lighter weight for residents with muscle weakness[13];

- For the resident who has the use of only one hand: holders for kitchen items, magazines/books, playing cards; items (e.g., art work, bingo card, nail file) taped to the table; c-clamp or suction vise to hold wood for sanding;

- For the resident with cognitive impairment: task segmentation and simplification; programs using retained long-term memory, rather than short-term memory; length of activities based on attention span; settings that recreate past experiences or increase/decrease stimulation; smaller groups without interruption; one-to-one activities;

NOTE: The length, duration, and content of specific one-to-one activities are determined by the specific needs of the individual resident, such as several short interventions (rather than a few longer activities) if someone has extremely low tolerance, or if there are behavioral issues. Examples of one-to-one activities may include any of the following:

  o Sensory stimulation or cognitive therapy (e.g., touch/visual/auditory stimulation, reminiscence, or validation therapy) such as special stimulus rooms or equipment; alerting/upbeat music and using alerting aromas or providing fabrics or other materials of varying textures;

  o Social engagement (e.g., directed conversation, initiating a resident to resident conversation, pleasure walk or coffee visit);

  o Spiritual support, nurturing (e.g., daily devotion, Bible reading, or prayer with or for resident per religious requests/desires);

  o Creative, task-oriented activities (e.g., music or pet activities/ therapy, letter writing, word puzzles); or

  o Support of self-directed activity (e.g., delivering of library books, craft material to rooms, setting up talking book service).

- For the resident with a language barrier: translation tools; translators; or publications and/or audio/video materials in the resident's language;

- For residents who are terminally ill: life review; quality time with chosen relatives, friends, staff, and/or other residents; spiritual support; touch; massage; music; and/or reading to the resident; [8]

NOTE: Some residents may prefer to spend their time alone and introspectively. Their refusal of activities does not necessarily constitute noncompliance.

- For the resident with pain: spiritual support, relaxation programs, music, massage, aromatherapy, pet therapy/pet visits, and/or touch;

- For the resident who prefers to stay in her/his own room or is unable to leave her/his room: in-room visits by staff/other residents/volunteers with similar interests/hobbies; touch and sensory activities such as massage or aromatherapy; access to art/craft materials, cards, games, reading materials; access to technology of interest (computer, DVD, hand held video games, preferred radio programs/stations, audio books); and/or visits from spiritual counselors; 14

- For the resident with varying sleep patterns, activities are available during awake time. Some facilities use a variety of options when activities staff are not available for a particular resident: nursing staff reads a newspaper with resident; dietary staff makes finger foods available; CNA works puzzle with the resident; maintenance staff take the resident on night rounds; and/or early morning delivery of coffee/juice to residents;

- For the resident who has recently moved-in: welcoming activities and/or orientation activities;

- For the short-stay resident: "a la carte activities" are available, such as books, magazines, cards, word puzzles, newspapers, CDs, movies, and handheld games; interesting/contemporary group activities are offered, such as dominoes, bridge, Pinochle, poker, video games, movies, and travelogues; and/or individual activities designed to match the goals of therapy, such as jigsaw puzzles to enhance fine motor skills;

- For the younger resident: individual and group music offerings that fit the resident's taste and era; magazines, books and movies that fit the resident's taste and era; computer and Internet access; and/or contemporary group activities, such as video games, and the opportunity to play musical instruments, card and board games, and sports; and

- For residents from diverse ethnic or cultural backgrounds: special events that include meals, decorations, celebrations, or music; visits from spiritual leaders and other individuals of the same ethnic background; printed materials (newspapers, magazines) about the resident's culture; and/or opportunities for the resident and family to share information about their culture with other residents, families, and staff.

Activity Approaches for Residents with Behavioral Symptoms [15, 7]

When the surveyor is evaluating the activities provided to a resident who has behavioral symptoms, they may observe that many behaviors take place at about the same time every day (e.g., before lunch or mid-afternoon). The facility may have identified a resident's pattern of behavior symptoms and may offer activity interventions, whenever possible, prior to the behavior occurring. Once a behavior escalates, activities may be less effective or may even cause further stress to the resident (some behaviors may be appropriate reactions to feelings of discomfort, pain, or embarrassment, such as aggressive behaviors exhibited by some residents with dementia during bathing [16]). Examples of activities-related interventions that a facility may provide to try to minimize distressed behavior may include, but are not limited to the following:

For the resident who is constantly walking:

- Providing a space and environmental cues that encourages physical exercise, decreases exit behavior and reduces extraneous stimulation (such as seating areas spaced along a walking path or garden; a setting in which the resident may manipulate objects; or a room with a calming atmosphere, for example, using music, light, and rocking chairs);

- Providing aroma(s)/aromatherapy that is/are pleasing and calming to the resident; and

- Validating the resident's feelings and words; engaging the resident in conversation about who or what they are seeking; and using one-to-one activities, such as reading to the resident or looking at familiar pictures and photo albums.

For the resident who engages in name-calling, hitting, kicking, yelling, biting, sexual behavior, or compulsive behavior:

- Providing a calm, non-rushed environment, with structured, familiar activities such as folding, sorting, and matching; using one-to-one activities or small group activities that comfort the resident, such as their preferred music, walking quietly with the staff, a family member, or a friend; eating a favorite snack; looking at familiar pictures;

- Engaging in exercise and movement activities; and

- Exchanging self-stimulatory activity for a more socially-appropriate activity that uses the hands, if in a public space.

For the resident who disrupts group activities with behaviors such as talking loudly and being demanding, or the resident who has catastrophic reactions such as uncontrolled crying or anger, or the resident who is sensitive to too much stimulation:

- Offering activities in which the resident can succeed, that are broken into simple steps, that involve small groups or are one-to-one activities such as using the computer, that are short and repetitive, and that are stopped if the resident becomes overwhelmed (reducing excessive noise such as from the television);

- Involving in familiar occupation-related activities. (A resident, if they desire, can do paid or volunteer work and the type of work would be included in the resident's plan of care, such as working outside the facility, sorting supplies, delivering resident mail, passing juice and snacks, refer to F169, Work);

- Involving in physical activities such as walking, exercise or dancing, games or projects requiring strategy, planning, and concentration, such as model building, and creative programs such as music, art, dance or physically resistive activities, such as kneading clay, hammering, scrubbing, sanding, using a punching bag, using stretch bands, or lifting weights; and

- Slow exercises (e.g., slow tapping, clapping or drumming); rocking or swinging motions (including a rocking chair).

For the resident who goes through others' belongings:

- Using normalizing activities such as stacking canned food onto shelves, folding laundry; offering sorting activities (e.g., sorting socks, ties or buttons); involving in organizing tasks (e.g., putting activity supplies away); providing rummage areas in plain sight, such as a dresser; and

- Using non-entry cues, such as "Do not disturb" signs or removable sashes, at the doors of other residents' rooms; providing locks to secure other resident's belongings (if requested).

For the resident who has withdrawn from previous activity interests/customary routines and isolates self in room/bed most of the day:

- Providing activities just before or after meal time and where the meal is being served (out of the room);

- Providing in-room volunteer visits, music, or videos of choice;

- Encouraging volunteer-type work that begins in the room and needs to be completed outside of the room, or a small group activity in the resident's room, if the resident agrees; working on failure-free activities, such as simple structured crafts or other activity with a friend; having the resident assist another person;

- Inviting to special events with a trusted peer or family/friend;

- Engaging in activities that give the resident a sense of value (e.g., intergenerational activities that emphasize the resident's oral history knowledge);

- Inviting resident to participate on facility committees;

- Inviting the resident outdoors; and

- Involving in gross motor exercises (e.g., aerobics, light weight training) to increase energy and uplift mood.

For the resident who excessively seeks attention from staff and/or peers: Including in social programs, small group activities, service projects, with opportunities for leadership.

For the resident who lacks awareness of personal safety, such as putting foreign objects in her/his mouth or who is self-destructive and tries to harm self by cutting or hitting self, head banging, or causing other injuries to self:

- Observing closely during activities, taking precautions with materials (e.g., avoiding sharp objects and small items that can be put into the mouth);

- Involving in smaller groups or one-to-one activities that use the hands (e.g., folding towels, putting together PVC tubing);

- Focusing attention on activities that are emotionally soothing, such as listening to music or talking about personal strengths and skills, followed by participation in related activities; and

- Focusing attention on physical activities, such as exercise.

For the resident who has delusional and hallucinatory behavior that is stressful to her/him:

- Focusing the resident on activities that decrease stress and increase awareness of actual surroundings, such as familiar activities and physical activities; offering verbal reassurance, especially in terms of keeping the resident safe; and acknowledging that the resident's experience is real to her/him.

The outcome for the resident, the decrease or elimination of the behavior, either validates the activity intervention or suggests the need for a new approach.

ENDNOTES

[1] Miller, M. E., Peckham, C. W., & Peckham, A. B. (1998). Activities keep me going and going (pp. 217-224). Lebanon, OH: Otterbein Homes.

[2] Alzheimer's Association (n.d.). Activity based Alzheimer care: Building a therapeutic program.
Training presentation made 1998.

[3] Thomas, W. H. (2003). Evolution of Eden. In A. S. Weiner & J. L. Ronch (Eds.), Culture change in long-term care (pp. 146-157). New York: Haworth Press.

[4] Bowman, C. S. (2005). Living Life to the Fullest: A match made in OBRA '87. Milwaukee, WI: Action Pact, Inc.

[5] Glantz, C. G., & Richman, N. (2001). Leisure activities. In Occupational therapy: Practice skills for physical dysfunction. St Louis: Mosby.

[6] Glantz, C. G., & Richman, N. (1996). Evaluation and intervention for leisure activities, ROTE: Role of Occupational Therapy for the Elderly (2nd ed., p. 728). Bethesda, MD.: American Occupational Therapy Association.

[7] Glantz, C.G., & Richman, N. (1998). Creative methods, materials and models for training trainers in alzheimer's education (pp. 156-159). Riverwoods, IL: Glantz/Richman Rehabilitation Associates.

[8] Hellen, C. (1992). Alzheimer's disease: Activity-focused care (pp. 128-130). Boston, MA: Andover.

[9] American Occupational Therapy Association. (2002). Occupational therapy practice framework: domain & process. American Journal of Occupational Therapy, 56(6), 616-617. Bethesda, MD: American Occupational Therapy Association.

[10] Henderson, A., Cermak, S., Costner, W., Murray, E., Trombly, C., & Tickle-Gegnen, L. (1991). The issue is: Occupational science is multidimensional. American Journal of Occupational Therapy, 45, 370-372, Bethesda, MD: American Occupational Therapy Association.

[11] Pedretti, L. W. (1996). Occupational performance: A model for practice in physical dysfunction. In L.W. Pedretti (Ed.), Occupational therapy: Practice skills for physical dysfunction (4th ed., pp. 3-11). St. Louis: Mosby-Year Book

[12] Christenson, M. A. (1996). Environmental design, modification, and adaptation, ROTE: Role of occupational therapy for the elderly (2nd ed., pp. 380-408). Bethesda, MD: American Occupational Therapy Association.

[13] Coppard, B. M., Higgins, T., & Harvey, K.D. (2004). Working with elders who have orthopedic conditions. In S. Byers-Connon, H.L. Lohman, and R.L. Padilla (Eds.), Occupational therapy with elders: Strategies for the COTA (2nd ed., p. 293). St. Louis, MO: Elservier Mosby.

[14] Glantz, C. G., & Richman, N. (1992). Activity programming for the resident with mental illness (pp. 53-76). Riverwoods, IL: Glantz/Richman Rehabilitation Associates.

[15] Day, K., & Calkins, M. P. (2002). Design and dementia. In R. B. Bechtel & A. Churchman (Eds.), Handbook of environmental psychology (pp. 374-393). New York: Wiley.

[16] Barrick, A. L., Rader, J., Hoeffer, B., & , P. (2002). Bathing without a battle: Personal care of individuals with dementia (p. 4). New York: Springer.

Documentation in a S N A P
For Activity Programs
For Dietary Services
For Social Services

This set of easy reference books will provide you with valuable proven guidelines to help you with documentation skills to meet OBRA regulations and improve quality of care.

CONTENT

Rules for Recording
Resident Rights
MDS
Care Plan Terminology
Guidelines for Progress Notes
Quality Assessment Tools
Resident Council
Discharge Planning

> **Ten chapters with regulations, interpretive guidelines, sample forms and examples of terminology**

Quantity	Item	Price
	Documentation in a SNAP for Activity Programs 3rd Revision	$38.95
	Documentation in a SNAP for Dietary Services	$28.95
	Documentation in a SNAP for Social Services	$39.95

ORDER FORM

Orders must be prepaid. Add $4.00 for postage and handling. Allow 4 weeks for delivery
In California include 7.75% sales tax ($3.02). Make checks payable to SNAP
Mail Orders to: SNAP, PO Box 574, San Anselmo, CA 94979

Deliver to:_____ Telephone No._____

Facility Name:_____

Address:_____

City/State/Zip Code_____ACT